Books are to be returned on or before
the last date below

(555)

The Development of
Anaesthetic Apparatus

The Development of Anaesthetic Apparatus

A HISTORY BASED ON THE CHARLES KING COLLECTION
OF THE ASSOCIATION OF ANAESTHETISTS OF
GREAT BRITAIN AND IRELAND
BY K. BRYN THOMAS, F.F.A., R.C.S. (Eng)
Curator, Charles King Collection
Consultant Anaesthetist, Royal Berkshire Hospital, Reading

PUBLISHED FOR THE

ASSOCIATION OF ANAESTHETISTS OF

GREAT BRITAIN AND IRELAND BY

BLACKWELL SCIENTIFIC PUBLICATIONS

OXFORD LONDON EDINBURGH MELBOURNE

© 1975 by Blackwell Scientific Publications
Editorial offices:
Osney Mead, Oxford OX2 0EL
8 John Street, London WC1N 2ES
9 Forrest Road, Edinburgh EH1 2QH
214 Berkeley Street, Carlton
    Victoria 3053, Australia

First published 1975
Reprinted 1980

Printed and bound in Great Britain by
Whitefriars Press Ltd,
London and Tonbridge

DISTRIBUTORS

USA
    Blackwell Mosby Book Distributors
    11830 Westline Industrial Drive
    St Louis, Missouri 63141

Canada
    Blackwell Mosby Book Distributors
    86 Northline Road, Toronto
    Ontario, M4B 3E5

Australia
    Blackwell Scientific Book Distributors
    214 Berkeley Street, Carlton
    Victoria 3053

ISBN 0–632–00177–1

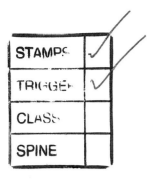
Contents

Foreword

L. RENDELL-BAKER

Professor and Chairman
Department of Anesthesiology
Mount Sinai School of Medicine of
the City University of New York

As the anaesthetist's best clinical efforts can so easily be frustrated by simple malfunction of apparatus, I am sure that there will be a wide-spread welcome for this fascinating review by Dr K. Bryn Thomas which brings to life the pioneers who designed the apparatus collected with such foresight by A. Charles King during the formative years of our specialty.

It is interesting to read how the tide of innovation swept back and forth across the North Atlantic and how the seed of many a brilliant idea failed to germinate due to the unsuitable soil in its homeland only to flourish in a more fertile foreign clime.

Wells and Morton, the American originators, respectively, of nitrous oxide and ether anaesthesia, had little personal success with their discoveries; Wells committed suicide and Morton took up farming in disgust at the lack of recognition for his discovery. Yet, in Britain, physicians and pharmacists enthusiastically studied the actions of ether and other agents evolving scientific apparatus for their safer use. In London, from these early days, succeeding generations of physicians built successful practices by devoting their professional energies to the administration of anaesthetics. But in the land of its origin this was not so, for the discovery of ether anaesthesia coincided with a 500 per cent increase in the land available for settlement following the purchase of Louisiana and the Mississippi Valley from France and the accession from Mexico of the future states of California, New Mexico, Nevada, Utah, Arizona, Wyoming, and Colorado. When gold was discovered soon thereafter in California, the 'gold-rush fever' of 1849 led to a surge of population to the West Coast which included Colton and many other physicians. This exodus of medical manpower from the East Coast states (which still continues in the 1970's), and the social restlessness of the times, were scarcely conducive to careful clinical or scientific development of anaesthesia, so that the simplest method—the ether sponge—administered by the most junior house staff or whoever else could be pressed into service, had to suffice.

In the 1860's, following the upheaval of the Civil War, construction of the trans-continental railways provided easy access to this vast empty space, comparable in size in Europe to all the land between the Straits of Dover and the Don River Basin in Russia. Into this population vacuum flowed not only settlers but more medical talent from the East. These physicians, already overworked, coping with the medical and surgical problems of masses of people on the move, depended on simple rudimentary anaesthesia given by any available helper.

By comparison, London in 1846 had enjoyed thirty years of peace since the defeat of Napoleon, which, with short interruptions in the Crimea, and in South Africa in 1901, was to last for a total of 99 years. London was fortunate to have a succession of medical men like Snow, Clover, Hewitt, Magill, and Rowbotham amongst others, interested in the mechanical and physiological aspects of anaesthetics, who were able to devote their time to the practice, study and teaching of anaesthesia. Within a year of ether's discovery, Snow's text *On the Inhalation of Ether* appeared in London to be followed in 1858 by his final work, *On Chloroform and Other Anaesthetics*.

Dr Bryn Thomas recounts how Colton's successful introduction of nitrous oxide for dentistry in New York in 1862 and its demonstration in London by Evans and Colton in 1868 led Clover to design an apparatus for its use as an induction agent before ether and the later refinement by Hewitt of an apparatus for nitrous oxide–oxygen anaesthesia. The description of his apparatus and methods in his text book on *Anaesthetics and Their Administration* by Hewitt in 1893, and the availability of both gases compressed in cylinders led to a new wave of technical development in the United States led by dentists like S.S.White, Teter, and Heidbrink, who introduced improved apparatus to utilize the methods Hewitt advocated. When Boothby and Colton added the bubble flowmeter, this provided, for the first time, visual evidence of the mixture delivered. The demonstration by Gwathmey in London in 1912 of his machine incorporating these flowmeters led Boyle to obtain a Gwathmey machine which served as a model for machines made for the British Army during World War I, to become known as Boyle machines. After fifty years of development and refinement had changed it beyond recognition, the tide of innovation carried the Boyle machine back across the Atlantic where U.S. manufacturers were influenced to adopt its modular construction and incidentally, its lay-out. This lay-out, with the flowmeters on the left, and the outlet to the patient on the right, was designed by Boyle for convenient use of the machine on his left hand side, as he was left handed.

Another innovation which bloomed abroad was the clinical use of cuffed endotracheal and endobronchial tubes. Though introduced into anaesthetic practice by Waters in the United States, they were developed by Magill and subsequent anaesthetists in Britain into a complete armamentarium to which was later added the Swedish Carlens double lumen bronchospirometric tube. Many variations of endobronchial and double lumen tubes were developed and are often used in Britain whereas they are but infrequently used in the United States.

Again, curare was introduced to 'soften' the contractions of electroconvulsion therapy by Bennett in the United States and as an adjunct to anaesthesia by Griffiths in Canada during World War II. However, it was in Liverpool that its full potential was exploited by Gray and colleagues to permit the use of extremely light nitrous oxide anaesthesia. The migration of British trained anaesthetists to North America has been followed by the use of apnoeic doses of curare, the routine use of controlled ventilation, and a veritable wave of automatic ventilators.

As an example of an American innovation which flourished in America but fell on stony ground abroad may be cited the failure of Hingson's technique of continuous caudal analgesia to be adopted in Britain in the late 1940's. No doubt this was due to a combination of conservative obstetricians and a shortage of anaesthetists interested in obstetrical anaesthesia. Later, in the 1960's British anaesthetists, after visits to U.S. centers, successfully introduced continuous epidural analgesia to a now more progressive generation of obstetricians and obstetrical patients.

Unfortunately, since 1962, the Food and Drug Administration regulations have made it very difficult for pharmacological tides of innovation to reach the shores of American clinical practice. With the imminence of further Federal regulations designed to ensure the safety and efficacy of medical devices, the possibility exists either for rapid improvement in these aspects, or the erection of further breakwaters against the innovative tides which enrich our clinical practice, with the hazard of stultification and inhibition of any except mandated changes.

This book will give the many who have been unable to examine this valuable collection of apparatus firsthand, the opportunity to do so at leisure guided by the curator. It is clear that progress requires not only brilliant conceptual seeds but also a fertile soil in which to grow. Dr Bryn Thomas has resurrected for us the giants of our past who so carefully nurtured the now fruitful garden of anaesthesia. Long may it flourish.

Preface

This work arose as a request from Council of the Association of Anaesthetists of Great Britain and Ireland that the inventory of the Charles King Collection of early anaesthetic apparatus, which was printed in 1970[1], should be amplified. In agreeing to Council's request, I stated that such an extension would probably transform itself into a book on the history and development of the apparatus, and this indeed has taken place. Though no claim is made that it is comprehensive, I have endeavoured to compare the collection specimens with their contemporaries (often from other countries) which are not represented in the collection. Brief historical introductions to the various sections also seemed essential to complete the perspective. These vary considerably in length, but I have discussed in greater detail some of those aspects of the anaesthesia story which do not appear in the textbooks, such as general analgesia and mixtures. Similarly, it was thought unnecessary to give space to long biographical notes of well-known pioneers such as Morton or Snow; lesser known physician-anaesthetists have been introduced in such detail as I have found available.

Considerations of time and space have also induced me to include in this volume only apparatus connected with inhalation. The Charles King Collection includes small and incomplete sections, for example, of gags and reducing valves; it would be audacious to produce a history of the laryngoscope from the only specimen available (no. Aust. 3).

As has been previously explained[1], the numbering of the collection is roughly, but not entirely, chronological, while the section bearing the numbers Aust 1–20 represents those items which were generously presented after the War to the Association by the then Australian Society of Anaesthetists.

In the present work, the items have been taken in sections representing the drug or function for which they were used, irrespective of their collection numbers, though the chronology has been maintained within the sections. For brevity, the numbers are preceded by CKC, for Charles King Collection, and Australian numbers by A.

In acknowledging those anaesthetists who have kindly donated items since the publication of the inventory, I must also record my awareness of the absence of post-war specimens in my survey. Since going to press, however, the Collection has been greatly improved by the donation of the British Oxygen Company's specimens, many of which are of late date. It has not been possible to include descriptions of these in the present work.

A collection such as this can only serve its full purpose if it is kept up-to-date; today's masterpiece is tomorrow's museum piece; but the time between 'today' and 'tomorrow' may be very short, and the 'masterpiece' may be an important link which should not be lost. The Charles King Collection is ready to receive any such items.

I wish to express my thanks to Council of the Association of Anaesthetists of Great Britain and Ireland, and to Dr John Beard, Dr Alfred Lee and Dr Philip Helliwell, successive Presidents of the Association, for their encouragement during the book's lengthy gestation, and for making publication possible.

Dr Beard was also responsible for persuading Council to finance the building of the new cabinets in which the collection is now on display, and for which Professor J.P.Payne has very generously allowed space in the Faculty Research Department of Anaesthetics at the Royal College of Surgeons of England; and here I must acknowledge the cabinet making skill of Mr Sidney Astill, senior technician to the department, and his assistant Mr Michael

Woods. I am also most grateful to Dr Douglas Howat, treasurer of the Association, and to my colleague at this hospital, Dr Tom Boulton, editor of *Anaesthesia*, for their constant encouragement.

I also acknowledge with much gratitude two friends without whom the book could not have been finished: Mrs Una Spanner who typed the original script, enduring the vagaries, inconsistencies and handwriting of its author over a period of several years; and Mr Lionel Williams of the Photographic Department, Royal Berkshire Hospital, for his skill and unfailing interest.

I must also thank the editorial and typographical staff of Blackwell Scientific Publications for making easy what seemed at the outset a formidable task.

The sources of the illustrations are listed, and I express my thanks to editors and publishers who readily gave permission for the reproduction of both illustrations and quotations. It will be seen that I have leaned heavily upon Barbara Duncum's classic monograph of 1947 and I am grateful to the Well-come Trustees for permission to quote her and to use her illustrations.

The photograph of Dr Minnitt was kindly provided by Professor Cecil Gray: that of Louis Ombrédanne by Professor Guy Vourc'h, who obtained the references: Mr Patrick Sim, Curator of the Wood Library/Museum, Chicago, has provided much information: I gratefully acknowledge also the help of other friends and colleagues who so readily responded to my requests for information, and especially to Professor Rendell-Baker, who not only answered my questions, but kindly and riskily agreed to write a foreword before he had even seen the text.

Finally I would acknowledge most humbly all those patients who trustingly and unconsciously have assisted anaesthetists throughout all these years.

Royal Berkshire Hospital   K. Bryn Thomas.
Reading
April 1975

REFERENCE

1 THOMAS, K.B. (1970) The A. Charles King Collection of early anaesthetic apparatus. *Anaesthesia* **25**, 548–564.

Section I
Ether Apparatus

ILLUSTRATIONS

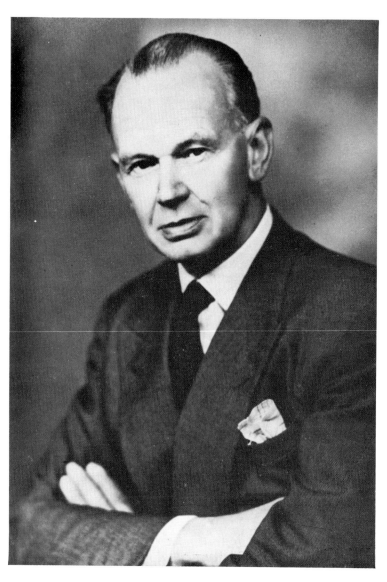

Arthur Charles King 1888–1966
Founder of the anaesthetics
equipment firm which bore his
name. Collector and annotator of
the early apparatus presented by
him in 1953 to the Association of
Anaesthetists of Great Britain and
Ireland. The Collection is now
housed at the Royal College of
Surgeons of England.

FIG. 1.1. WILLIAM THOMAS
GREEN MORTON 1819–1868
Dentist in Boston, Massachusetts.
On 16 October 1846 Morton gave
the first successful public
demonstration of ether anaesthesia
at the Massachusetts General
Hospital, John Collins Warren
being the surgeon. Anaesthesia
became rapidly established and
therefore to Morton belongs the
credit of its introduction.

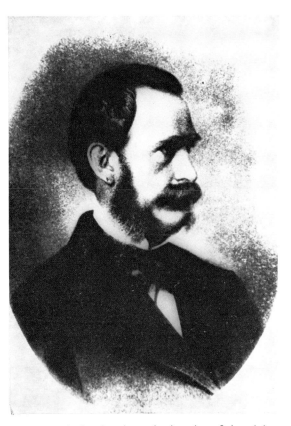

INTRODUCTION: *MORTON TO MACINTOSH*

When William Thomas Green Morton (Fig. 1.1) gave the first public demonstration of ether anaesthesia at the Massachusetts General Hospital on 16 October 1846 (Fig. 1.2) he used an apparatus of his own designing. Four years earlier Crawford Williamson Long had 'used the corner of a towel' to give ether to James Venable[1]. Various inhalers had been employed in previous years for the inhalation of medicants, and apparatus had been described by Humphry Davy at the Bristol Pneumatic Institute in 1799 for the inhalation of nitrous oxide. Ether itself had long been recommended for inhalation in various diseases such as asthma, but cautions were added against overdosage since the result of imprudence had been observed in the production of lethargic states; such observations were not followed up. The *Edinburgh Dispensatory* of 1786 stated that 'ether will give relief to violent headache by external application, and has been given internally with benefit in whooping cough, hysterical cases and asthma.' Morton had evidently experimented with various types of inhaler for we know that he sought help from the instrument maker Joseph Wightman, who wrote '. . . I consented to arrange a temporary apparatus. This was composed of a quart tubulated globe receiver, having a cork fitted into it instead of a glass stopper, through which cork a pipette was inserted to supply the ether as it evaporated. I then cut several large grooves around the cork to admit the air freely into the globe, to mix with the vapour.' Morton did not use this apparatus, but one which was described by H.J.Bigelow a few days after the first public use. Bigelow wrote, 'A small two-necked glass globe contains the prepared vapor, together with sponges to enlarge the evaporating surface. One

aperture admits the air to the interior of the globe, whence, charged with vapor it is drawn through the second into the lungs. The inspired air thus passes through the bottle but the expiration is diverted by a valve in the mouth piece and escaping into the apartment is thus prevented from vitiating the medicated vapor'[2]. This is recognizably the Morton inhaler. The Charles King replica (see p. 10) is based on this description and on the apparatus preserved at the Massachusetts General Hospital, which

FIG. 1.2. THE OLD OPERATING
THEATRE
Under the 'ether dome',
Massachusetts General Hospital,
scene of Morton's successful
demonstration.

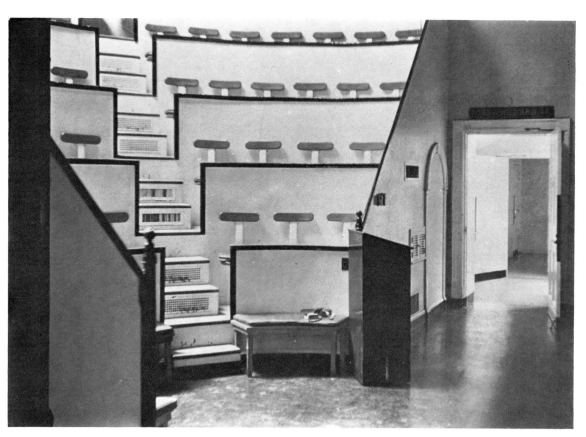

is said to be the one used by Morton himself.

When the news crossed the Atlantic, English doctors turned to the adaptation of existing apparatus and the invention of new. Thus William Squire, who was anaesthetist for the first major operation in London, at University College Hospital on 19 November 1846, used a Nooth's apparatus (a specimen of which may be seen at the Museum of the History of Science, Oxford), designed for the production of 'carbonic water'[3]. John Snow, on the other hand, designed his own apparatus from the first, and the description and drawing given in his book *On Ether*[4] is the origin of the specimen (Fig. 1.7) which Charles King had made in his own workshop. It is of some interest that the craftsman failed to follow Snow's description which stipulated that the spiral baffle should be soldered to the top of the circular ether chamber, and reach to one sixteenth of an inch from the bottom (see p. 13). The Charles King Collection specimen does not allow this space, the spiral being soldered above and below. The vaporizer is therefore unable to function.

Morton himself gave up the use of formal apparatus within a matter of months, and saw fit to write to the *Lancet* on this subject on 30 June 1847. This letter does not appear to have been noted previously, perhaps because the title is given merely as *Letter from Dr Morton:* he wrote

I take the liberty of stating to you an improvement I have made in the mode of administering ether in my practice, since my discovery was promulgated to the world. As in everything else new, I had to find my way along slowly and cautiously, after discovering the new property of ether, and was for some time greatly embarrassed in procuring a suitable apparatus. My first attempts were made with a sponge; next, I used a simple conical glass tube, with a sponge in the larger end; and after that, other instruments, none of which, however, affording but partial success.

Up to this time, I had given the ether but once at the Massachusetts General Hospital, which was on the 16th of October, and having another engagement there for the next day, (the 17th) and my first application being but partially successful, I found that, in the meantime, I must procure some more perfect apparatus. Accordingly, I conversed with Dr A.A. Gould, a distinguished physician of Boston, (late on the night of the 16th), as to the best means of rendering my newly discovered agent available, when he rendered me important service in arriving at the valvular system now in use in this country. I had these valves introduced into a glass globe the next morning, before the hour of my engagement at the hospital,— at eleven o'clock,—when the fact of my discovery, for the time being, at least, was to be settled. I had passed a sleepless night. In the morning, before light, I aroused an instrument-maker, and superintended the

work; and when the hour came, I went almost with a feverish excitement to the hospital. Heretofore, with two or three exceptions, surgeons, physicians, and all, were incredulous; so that, as may be easily seen, my position was a most trying one. But, with my new apparatus, I went before the doctors—gave the ether —when the second capital operation was performed, this time with perfect success. But the result of the experiment of the 17th of October is before the world. And the apparatus thus constructed is still generally in use in this country, although I have since discovered a far more simple and perfect means of administering the vapour; hence the object of this communication.

I was never satisfied with any apparatus at all for the purpose of inhalation, there being so much repugnance to it. I was led, therefore, to make further experiments on this subject, which have resulted in an entire abandonment of my old inhaler, and the substitution of the sponge. This should be about the size of the open hand, or a little larger, and concave, to suit over the nose and mouth. The sponge is then thoroughly saturated with ether, applied to the nose and mouth, and, with the latter open, the patient directed to inhale as fully and freely as possible. In this way, I have found the result more sure and satisfactory, and the difficulty of inhalation very much reduced, or entirely removed. The most delicate or nervous females, or aged persons, as well as young children, are thus rapidly and almost imperceptibly narcotized, even before they are aware, as in some cases, that the administration has commenced. The beauty and importance of this means is its perfect simplicity. Formerly, many persons could not be induced to persevere; now I do not find any who cannot inhale the vapour without serious difficulty.

Believing that this is an important improvement— at least on the means employed in this country—to produce insensibility to pain, and even without knowing that the sponge may not have been long since generally used elsewhere, I venture to throw out the hint, trusting that it may be of some service to those

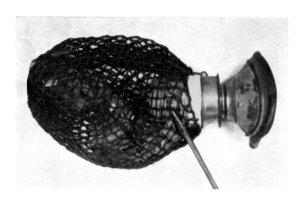

FIG. I.3. ORMSBY ETHER INHALER
1877
Lambert Hepenstal Ormsby, 1850–1923, surgeon of Dublin, described this inhaler in 1877, the same year as Clover introduced his portable regulating ether inhaler. Both were popular. The bag contained a small sponge in a wire cage.

who cannot readily get an inhaler, should one be preferred.—I am, respectfully, your obedient servant,
W.T.G.Morton

Boston, June 30th, 1847

* It is just to say, that the inhalation, by means of a sponge, had been recommended and practised for some time in this country, by Dr Smith, of Cheltenham.—Editor, *Lancet*'[5].

This important letter gives details of those two vital days in the history of anaesthesia which do not seem to have been correctly reported by subsequent historians.

The years following 1847 saw the introduction of chloroform, and the controversy of its use *vis-a-vis* ether. In spite of its reputation, even John Snow preferred its ease of use and action to that of ether. Before 1850 many forms of ether apparatus were designed, but for the next twenty-five years little was produced and the Charles King Collection reflects both this gap and the name of Clover in the next important phase of development of ether vaporizers.

In 1871, Hayward of St George's Hospital advocated the re-introduction of ether at a meeting of the Royal Medical and Chirurgical Society. Others were less enthusiastic; Clover stated that he had 'been in the habit of giving nitrous oxide first, and then ether, as the great difficulty was to get patients to inhale it freely'[6]. This was a reference to the first sequential nitrous oxide/ether apparatus, which Clover publicized in 1876. An original specimen is in the Collection (CKC 7, p. 121). The *British Medical Journal* threw its weight on the side of ether, chiefly on account of its greater safety, and very shortly ether began to oust chloroform for general use. Most surgeons and anaesthetists still used a sponge or towel, but Clover, with the inventive

mantle of Snow upon him, produced the gas/ether apparatus already mentioned (CKC 7) and the better known *Portable Regulating Ether Inhaler* of 1877 (CKC 8). Clover himself preferred the former apparatus, though the latter achieved more fame and was copied and modified by anaesthetists far and wide. Thus Wilson-Smith of Bath produced a large bore inhaler in 1899 (CKC 13): Probyn-Williams of the London Hospital similarly in 1908 (CKC 19) and, best known of all the large bore modifications, Hewitt's version of 1901 (CKC 16). On the Continent, Ombrédanne's inhaler of 1908 (CKC 47) resembled the Clover, though it allowed a small air entry. The Ombrédanne inhaler is possibly still in use in some areas. The Charles King Collection is fortunate in possessing all these types, which will be described in the following pages.

A natural improvement to this type of inhaler was its adaptation to the passage of nitrous oxide, described by Hewitt in his book[7]. Even more popular than the Clover was the inhaler described by Ormsby[8] of Dublin only a week or two after Clover's account. In 1893 Hewitt wrote 'For inducing anaesthesia by means of ether there is no apparatus which can be compared to that invented by Clover, for the anaesthetic vapour may be admitted so gradually that the initial discomforts are reduced to a minimum. But for *maintaining* ether anaesthesia Ormsby's inhaler is equal, and in many cases superior to Clover's'[9]. Unfortunately, the Charles King Collection does not possess an Ormsby inhaler (Fig. 1.3).

In the late 1870's 'open' ether masks began their long history; these are described in a later section. A later development of interest was the 'Pinson ether bomb' of 1921, which used a hitherto undeveloped idea of ether vapour under pressure produced by heating the container (CKC 35, Fig. 1.46).

FIG. I.4. OXFORD VAPORIZER 1941
A 'draw-over' apparatus with a
'non-rebreathing' concertina
reservoir bag. The ether chamber is
kept at a constant temperature
(30°C) by the melting and
recrystallization of hydrated
calcium chloride, the initial heat
being provided by boiling water
placed in a central chamber.
Concentrations up to 25 per cent
ether vapour may be obtained, but
no allowance is made for variations
due to respiratory rate or volume.
Specimen at the Royal Berkshire
Hospital, Reading.

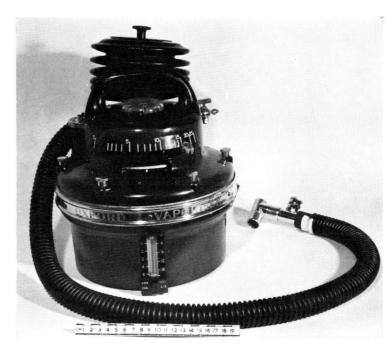

Yet another ingenious apparatus, not in the collection* was the Oxford Ether Vaporizer designed by Professor Macintosh and Dr Epstein in 1941[10] for service use. In this the ether compartment was heated by making use of the latent heat of crystallization of calcium chloride, itself heated by an inner chamber of hot water (Fig. 1.4).

In the meantime, however, the introduction of nitrous oxide and oxygen apparatus had allowed for ether vaporization by gaseous carriers. These types will be described under the heading of sequential apparatus.

* A specimen is now on loan to the Charles King Collection from the Anaesthetic Department, Frenchay Hospital, Bristol, by courtesy of Dr T.Wilton, FFARCS

CKC 1: MORTON ETHER INHALER
1846 (replica)

The replica (Fig. 1.5) was presented in 1950 by the New York State Society of Anesthesiologists. This is the 'small two-necked glass globe' described by Bigelow as used by Morton (see p. 5). It is 125mm in diameter and contains a sponge. The inhaling port is 20mm in internal diameter and the air inlet 30mm. Bigelow describes an expiratory valve and it is known that Morton designed such a valve of brass. This specimen has a wooden spigot with a tap, but no valve. Gwathmey[11] has a picture of 'The original Morton Inhaler' which clearly shows a similar spigot. The example in the possession of the

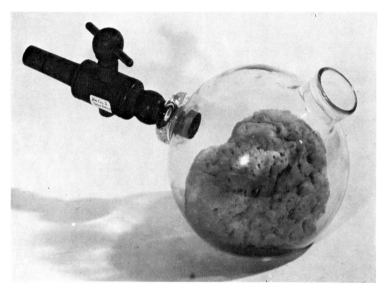

FIG. 1.5. MORTON ETHER INHALER
1846
Replica made in 1950 and presented
by the New York State Society of
Anesthesiologists to the Association
of Anaesthetists of Great Britain
and Ireland.
It is now suggested that this pattern,
with a wooden spigot, was the type
used for Morton's first public
demonstration on 16 October 1846.
By the following day he had
incorporated valves into a brass
mouth-piece inserted into the globe.
(Letter from Dr Morton, *Lancet*,
1847, **ii**, 80 see p. 7).
CKC I

Massachusetts General Hospital, Boston, has brass inspiratory and expiratory valves and is said to be the original used by Morton on 16 October 1846[12]. It seems from the letter of Morton to the *Lancet* (p. 7), that this type of apparatus with a valve was used only at the second operation on 17 October and was that described in Bigelow's paper. It is thus at least possible that the apparatus used for the first operation had a wooden spigot and no valve; this would certainly account for Morton's 'first application being but partially successful', as he himself wrote in that letter.

Morton's tragedy has been amply documented by Duncum[12] and many others[13]: but his prime position in anaesthesia was stated in the inscription written by Jacob Bigelow over his tomb in Mount Auburn Cemetery, Boston:

William T.G.Morton, Inventor and Revealer of anaesthetic inhalation, by whom pain in surgery was averted and annulled: before whom, in all times, surgery was agony; since whom, science has control of pain.

CKC 2: SNOW ETHER INHALER
1847 (replica)

John Snow 1813–1858[14, 15] (Fig. 1.6), the first specialist anaesthetist in the world, produced this apparatus within a few months of the introduction of ether (Fig. 1.7). The replica was made in 1950 by J.Hawkes for Charles King.

John Snow recognized the need for wide bore tubing, for adequate exposure of ether area, and for warming of the ether chamber. These needs he supplied, and he described his apparatus in early

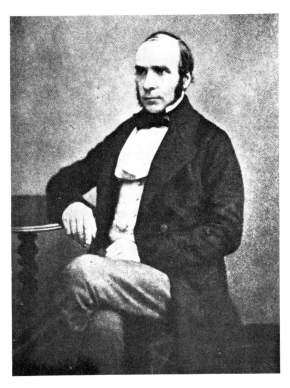

1847 in his book *On Ether*[16]. The drum-like metal ether chamber is 150mm in diameter and 35mm deep. It has two orifices, one central and one peripheral, the latter having a screw-on inlet tube 155mm long to prevent evaporation; of this Snow wrote 'it effects this object in a more simple manner than a valve would and offers less resistance than the most delicately balanced valve'. The drum contains a metal spiral baffle of five turns, which is soldered to the upper plate of the chamber and has a gap of one-sixteenth of an inch (1.5mm) between it and the bottom plate (Figs. 1.8, 1.9). Snow regarded these

dimensions as critical. He wrote[16] 'when an inspiration is taken, the air, having entered by this tube, which is five-eighths of an inch in internal diameter, passes round four times on the surface of the ether and becomes saturated with its vapour. . . . The dimensions of the ether chamber are not a matter of indifference. It is nearly six inches in diameter and an inch and a quarter in depth. . . . It is desirable to have the chamber as shallow as practicable, in order that all the air passing through it may be brought successively in contact with the surface of the ether: and on the other hand, it is necessary to leave a considerable space above the ether for the air: otherwise when a patient draws vigorous and deep inspirations the ether will be agitated into waves and splashed into the elastic tube. The space between the coils of the volute is five-eighths of an inch and it is important that it is uniformly turned.'

The drum stands in a rectangular water bath (acting also as a container for the whole) which, Snow wrote, 'holds above 100 cubic inches . . . (this) will supply the caloric necessary to the conversion of one or two ounces of ether into vapour without being much reduced in temperature. . . .'[17].

The tube as defined by Snow is three feet in length, and is designedly wider than the trachea, being three-quarters of an inch internally, 'to compensate for the resistance arising from frictions of the air against the interior of the tube.' 'The tube should be so capacious as to offer no impediment to the most rapid respiration', wrote Snow.

The face piece is a modification of that designed by Francis Sibson (1814–1876) of the General Hospital, Nottingham, and later of St Mary's Hospital, London. The central part containing the valves is of white metal and the remainder of thin sheet lead, covered with silk or glove-leather. 'The

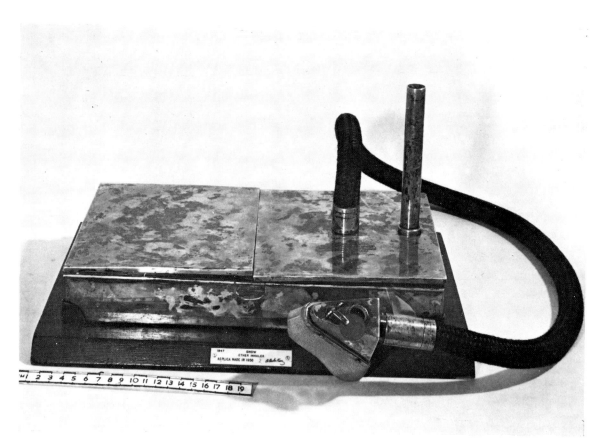

valves are of vulcanised India rubber. . . . I have contrived the expiratory valve to turn on a pivot so as to allow the admission of external air.' An inspiratory valve prevents rebreathing. Snow added a note that the apparatus had been made by Mr Ferguson, Mr Coxeter and others, and says 'there is no restriction respecting the making of it'[18].

FIG. I.7. SNOW ETHER INHALER 1847
Replica made in Charles King's workshop in 1950.
CKC 2

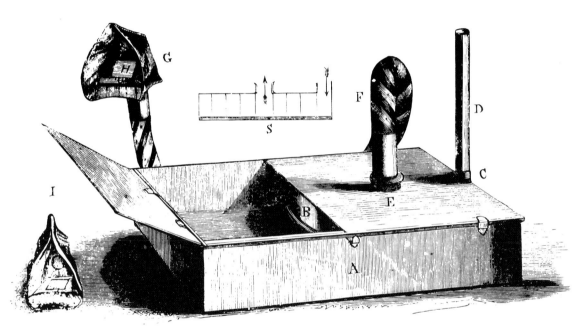

FIG. 1.8. SNOW ETHER INHALER showing inhaling tube and face piece, screw-on inlet tube *D* and scheme of baffle, which reaches to one-sixteenth inch (1.5mm) of the base of the ether drum *B*. From Snow, J. (1847) *On Ether*, p. 17.

FIG. 1.9. BAFFLE AND FACE PIECE
OF SNOW INHALER
From Snow, J. (1847) *On Ether*,
p. 18.

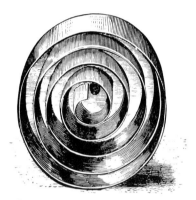

Drawing of ether chamber, with the bottom removed to shew the interior. The volute, of the same metal as the chamber, is soldered to the top, and reaches to one-sixteenth of an inch from the bottom.

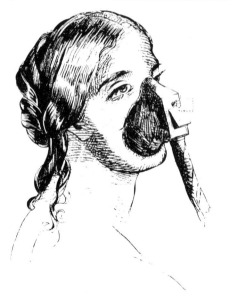

The dotted lines indicate the position of the expiratory valve when turned aside for the admission of unvaporized air.

CKC 8: CLOVER PORTABLE REGULATING ETHER INHALER 1877

Joseph Clover (1825–1882) (Fig. 1.10)[19] described this apparatus in 1877[20], and it became a very popular method of administration. It was the first to provide a convenient means of regulating the amount of vapour inhaled, and many anaesthetists wrote of the comparative ease of induction.

The ether container consists of a spherical metal chamber approximately 9cm in diameter; soldered to this is a closed tubular extension of the same diameter containing water, by means of which half of the chamber is insulated. The whole inhaler was sometimes warmed in hot water before use, and the heat of the hand, with the patient's exhalations, assisted in preventing cooling by evaporation. (Figs. 1.11, 1.12).

The ether chamber and water compartment together revolved upon a divided circular tube, approximately 13cm in length and 22mm in internal diameter, which was provided with ports separated in later models by a baffle. Clover's original description shows two 'whistle-tip' tubes (Fig. 1.13), which rotated relative to one another so that the 'whistle-tips' were aligned when the patient breathed directly from the bag, or were partly or completely separated, when a proportion of the respiration was diverted into the ether chamber. (Figs. 1.14 to 1.17). The later models were simplified to the single tube with ports and baffle as shown in the sectioned Charles King specimen (Fig. 1.11)[21].

The diameter of the control tube varies with the specimen, but the present item is of 22mm proximal and 25mm distal diameters. As half only was available the area used was 190sq mm. The whole apparatus, unfilled, weighs 1 lb 4oz (504g).

The chamber rotated upon the tube and control,

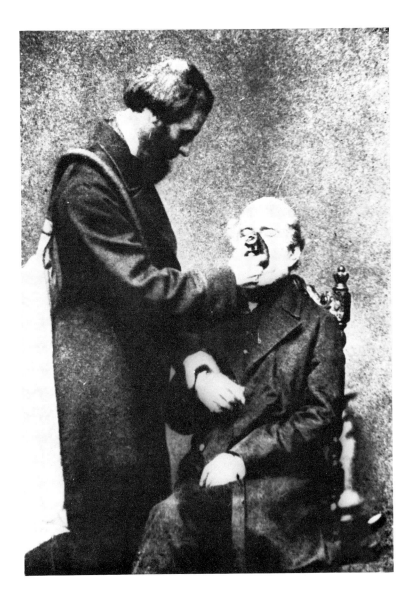

FIG. I.IO. JOSEPH THOMAS CLOVER administering 4 per cent chloroform in air to a patient. Clover used this bag also for nitrous oxide. A similar means of administration had been suggested by John Snow some years previously. Note the finger on the pulse.

FIG. I.II. SECTIONED CLOVER
PORTABLE REGULATING ETHER
INHALER.
The control tube from another is
also shown. Compare the design
with Figs. I.13 (earlier) and I.17
(similar internal arrangement of
ports). The earlier design had two
similar tubes of 'whistle-tip'
pattern, the tips being placed
end-to-end inside the outer tube.
This arrangement was found to
leak, and the single tube with ports
supplanted the 'whistle-tip' tubes.
CKC 8

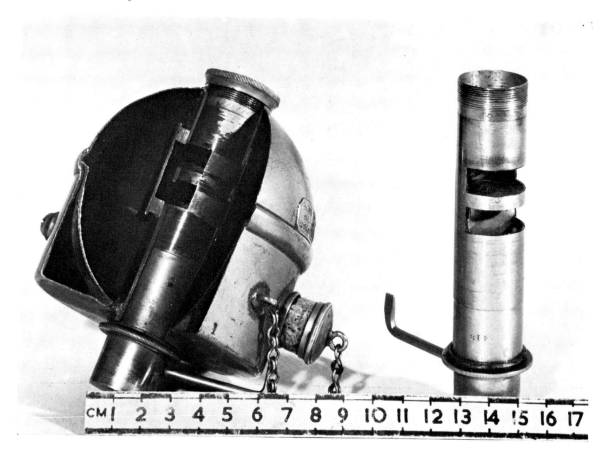

FIG. 1.12. COMPLETE CLOVER'S
INHALER
(with modern mask and bag). It is
noteworthy that Clover's
diameters (22mm) fit these modern
accessories.

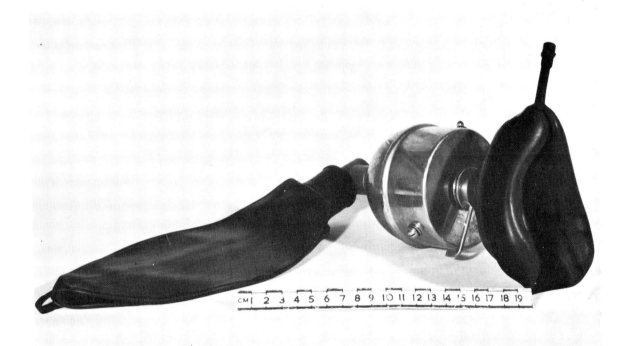

but this was inconvenient, and later developments, e.g. Hewitt's, allowed rotation of the control without rotating the chamber (Fig. 1.16). No air was admitted and Clover wrote 'the plan of excluding fresh air until insensibility has been induced and admitting it very sparingly afterwards, has now been extensively tried and is practically free from the danger of

causing obstruction to the pulmonary circulation and overdistension of the right cavities of the heart. Of course air cannot be indefinitely excluded, but the pulse and respiration give timely notice when air is required. A single artificial respiration of fresh air in these cases affords more relief than several such respirations when the apnoea has resulted from an

FIG. I.13. DIAGRAM OF CLOVER'S
ORIGINAL DESIGN
from his paper in *Brit. med. J.*
(1877), **i**, 69.
Note the 'whistle-tip' tubes, and
compare with the arrangement in
Figs. I.11, I.14, I.17.

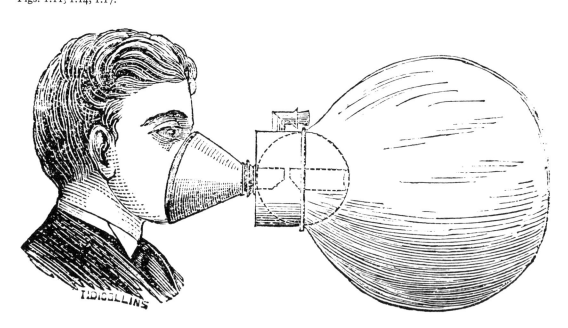

overdose of ether'[20].

Clover claimed the following advantages for his apparatus:

1   it has no valves;
2   it supplies the vapour so gradually that patients breathe quietly;
3   it produces sleep in two minutes;
4   it does not require fresh ether during the con-

tinuance of an operation;
5   the recovery from a short operation is more speedy than with most other inhalers;
6   it does not need to be warmed before use;
7   no sponge or felt is required;
8   ether left in the inhaler can be saved for another time.

FIG. I.I4. SCHEME OF SECTIONED
INHALER
in its original whistle-tip form. The
indicator *i* is at full, and all the
respired air passes into the ether
chamber. From Hewitt, F.W. (1893)
Anaesthetics, p. 141

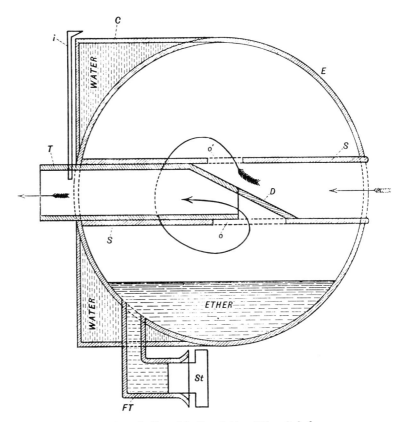

Section of Clover's Portable Regulating Ether Inhaler.

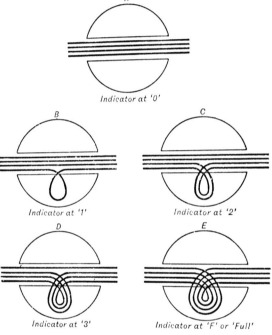

Indicator at '0'

Indicator at '1'   Indicator at '2'

Indicator at '3'   Indicator at 'F' or 'Full'

FIG. 1.15. SCHEME SHOWING
PASSAGE OF THE RESPIRED AIR
at different settings. From Hewitt,
F.W. (1893) *Anaesthetics*, p. 142

Diagram showing the extent to which the air-current passes over ether in Clover's Portable Inhaler when the indicator points to '0,' '1,' '2,' '3,' and 'F.' The whole current is diagramatically represented by four lines.

Clover had produced his nitrous oxide/ether apparatus (CKC 7, see p. 121) one year earlier, in 1876; he was thus aware of the advantages of a nitrous oxide induction followed by ether, and the *regulating* apparatus in many instances was so used, a full gas-bag being attached to the apparatus; re-breathing was then allowed until the patient was sufficiently unconscious to begin the introduction of ether. Hewitt used this method with the addition of his 'stopcock' (see Fig. 1.25). This had the great advantage that air could be admitted without raising the mask, and was the original of later and more highly developed Hewitt stopcocks (see CKC 12, p. 125).

Some of the many modifications and redesignings of Clover's regulating inhaler will be seen in the following pages, and an interesting paper by Charles King himself, with Dr Archibald Galley, refers in some detail to these important developments in ether anaesthesia[22].

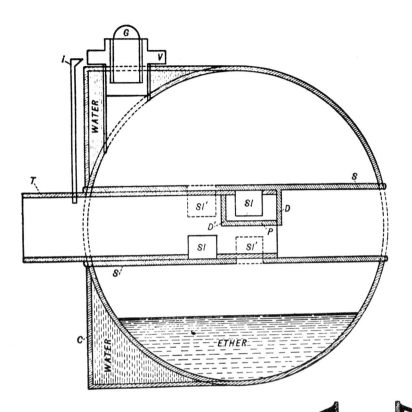

FIG. 1.16. ONE MODIFICATION
WHICH HEWITT
made was to alter the shape of the
central tube and parts. The reason
for this was to prevent leakage at
the bearing surface of the 'whistle-
tips'. The central tube rotated
inside a larger shaft.
From Hewitt,F.W. (1893)
Anaesthetics. p. 143

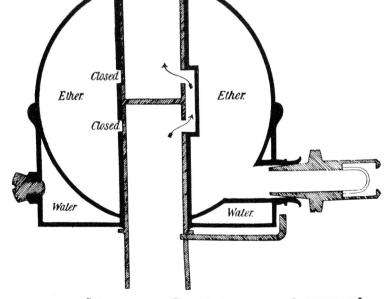

FIG. 1.17. A COMMON FORM OF
MODIFICATION
(cf. Fig. 1.13). Rotation of the ether
chamber causes the ports on the
central column to move either to
open into the ether chamber or to
close this and open directly via the
raised section, as shown.
From Probyn-Williams,R.J. (1909)
*A Practical Guide to the
Administration of Anaesthetics.*
p. 117.

SECTION THROUGH CLOVER'S INHALER WITH INDICATOR AT 0.
All the breath is passing through the column, from the face-piece to the bag and
back, without any entering the ether chamber

Rebreathing bag missing. Note the
similarity in shape to Clover's inhaler.
The control tube is of wide bore,
36mm in diameter (cf. Clover, 22mm)
but is reduced to half by the 'whistle-
tip' seen in Fig. 1.19.
CKC 13

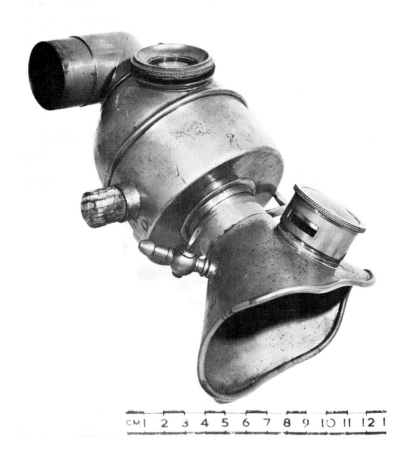

CKC 13: WILSON-SMITH ETHER INHALER 1899

Dr Thomas Wilson-Smith, 1864–1955, was consultant physician anaesthetist to the Royal United Hospitals, Bath[23]. A student and resident at Guy's Hospital, he was described as a man of 'dignified bearing and of culture'. His obituary notice does not mention any interest in anaesthesia.

The specimen of his inhaler is number 312303, manufactured by Mayer and Meltzer, and was presented by Dr Wilson-Smith himself (Fig. 1.18).

A.H.Galley and Charles King in their article of 1948[24] show that Wilson-Smith has a prior claim over Hewitt (1901) in the introduction of a 'wide-bore' inhaler, for he first described a modified

Clover inhaler in the *Lancet* of 1898[25]. This had channels of the same diameter as the original Clover but Wilson-Smith, one year later, described the present apparatus in which the bore area was equal to that of the trachea[26]. It is a curious fact that it took twenty-two years for anaesthetists to realize this particular limitation of the Clover inhaler, though many must have been aware of the need, which Snow had postulated in 1847. Wilson-Smith himself wrote 'Mayer and Meltzer have constructed for me an inhaler . . . with an airway throughout fully equal to the tracheal sectional area, i.e. double that of the ordinary Clover's inhaler, with the result that the sound of 'stridor' observable in the old apparatus is practically abolished, the breathing being quiet and 'breezy' in character'[27].

Wilson-Smith had examined the interior of a Clover inhaler, using a laryngoscopic mirror[28]. He found considerable corrosion, and described his new apparatus thus: 'In the dome of the ether chamber are two circular apertures into which are screwed two watch glasses . . . so that the quantity of ether can be seen at any time. To facilitate thorough cleansing and to afford a good light in the ether chamber, the interior (Fig. 1.19) surface is plated and polished in the same manner as the exterior.' The water-jacket had a detachable screw so that warm water could be introduced. Allowance was made for admission of air by means of a slotted metal cap in the distal end of the rebreathing bag, (not present on this specimen). (See E, Fig. 1.20).

The main body is similar in shape and dimensions to the original Clover (see p. 17). The face piece is of metal and would have had a rubber cushion. A

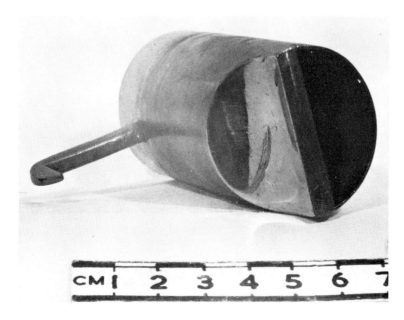

FIG. 1.19. CONTROL TUBE OF WILSON-SMITH INHALER to show 'whistle-tip' and indicator. As in the Clover inhaler, the ether chamber rotated upon the tube.

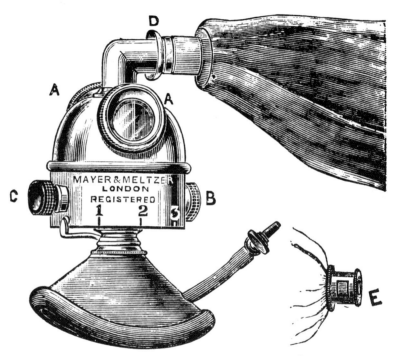

A, Windows looking into ether chamber. B, Stopper of
aperture for filling hot-water jacket. C, Stopper of aperture
for filling ether chamber. E, Air-opening into bag.

rubber expiratory valve on the face piece shows that gases were admitted, and a nitrous oxide tube with tap is fitted to the bag angle-piece to facilitate induction. A side tube with tap on the face piece is probably for oxygen. The rotating control tube is 77mm in length and 36mm bore, but the proximal opening is reduced to half (500sq mm) by a baffle. This tube is 'whistle-ended' and this meets another 'whistle-end' within the body of the ether chamber. A rectangular port within the tube is 16mm ×

30mm equalling 480sq mm (Clover's is 190sq mm). According to Galley and King, Wilson-Smith said his main reason for redesigning was to reduce weight, and that his inhaler weighed 6 oz (170 g) less than Clover's. Galley and King, however, found that it weighed 6 oz more. The present specimen weighs 1 lb 10 oz (728 g): the Clover weighs 1 lb 4 oz (504 g).

The Wilson-Smith inhaler was an improvement upon the Clover chiefly for its wide bore design. It

FIG. 1.21. SIR FREDERICK HEWITT, 1857–1916,
anaesthetist to Charing Cross
Hospital, inventor of apparatus,
writer and teacher. Known also for
administration of ether to King
Edward VII in 1902 for which he
used a Rendle ether inhaler.
See CKC 64

suffered from the same drawback that the chamber rotated upon the central tube. The Mayer and Meltzer model is a beautifully made piece of apparatus and there is no sign of corrosion in the silvered interior.

CKC 16: HEWITT ETHER INHALER 1901

Frederick Hewitt 1857–1916[29] (Fig. 1.21), described his inhaler in the second edition of his book *Anaesthetics*[30] (Fig. 1.22). His object was to avoid the difficulties arising from anoxia when using Clover's inhaler. Others confirmed this: for example Bellamy Gardner in 1916 mentioned the restricted size of the air-channels of the Clover 'and the comparatively weak anaesthetic effect which it produces without an undue limitation of the air supply, which renders the patient dusky in colour and produces venous oozing in the field of operation'[31]. Hewitt, however, made no particular provision for the admission of air, but he increased the diameter of his control tube to 31mm, and though baffles reduced this to half, the effective area was 377sq mm (cf. Clover, 190sq mm).

The control tube was divided into three parts, (Fig. 1.23) of 31mm, 32mm, and 23mm in length, each being baffled for half its area. The two outer portions were connected by a handle to rotate together within the central tube, while the middle portion (23mm long) was soldered to this central tube. Close to the fixed portion on either side two slots were cut into the ether compartment. These were 10mm wide and half the circumference in length (area approximately 500sq mm). When the tube baffles are arranged to alternate (i.e. when the control points to full ether) the breathed gases pass

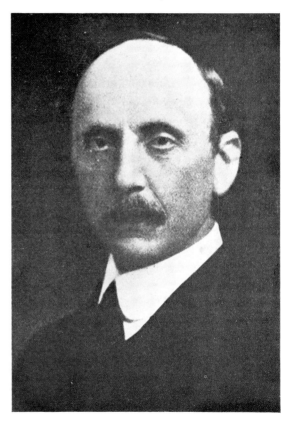

through these slots into the ether chamber and out again to the rebreathing bag. (see Fig. 1.24). The chamber is more ovoid than the Clover, thus lowering the centre of gravity in use; the water compartment, though present,* is small, (Hewitt recommended

* In my published inventory of the Charles King Collection (*Anaesthesia*, 1970, **25**, 555) it is stated that the water bath was omitted. This is not so. It was much reduced in size compared with the Clover (see Fig. 1.24). K.B.T.

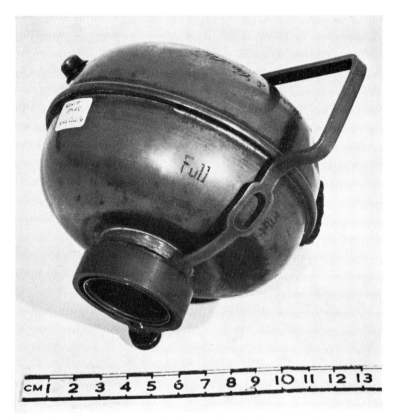

FIG. I.22. HEWITT WIDE BORE
ETHER INHALER, 1901.
Collar for mask is shown and the
bag is missing. The handle connects
the two outer segments of the
control tube, which thus rotate
together.
CKC 16

immersion in warm water before use) and there is a glass domed filler to allow inspection of the ether level. The recommended filling of ether was $1\frac{1}{2}$ oz (42ml) which would last ten to fifteen minutes. The water chamber is seen as an infolded segment in the sectioned specimen (Fig. I.24). It was suggested that air be admitted for every fifth inhalation, the mask being lifted for the purpose.

The inhaler was commonly used with a nitrous oxide induction sequence, when the gas was admitted from a two gallon bag, and Hewitt's stopcock allowed the controlled admission of air (see Fig I.25, and CKC 12, p. 125). When the patient was unconscious the two gallon nitrous oxide bag and stopcock were removed, a smaller rebreathing bag substituted, and maintenance continued with ether. Hewitt claimed that using this sequence 'stertor and cyanosis are lessened, and the patient passes smoothly, with little or no respiratory derangement from the anaesthetic of nitrous oxide to that of ether' [30.31].

FIG. I.23. CONTROL TUBE OF
HEWITT INHALER.
Showing the three baffled segments;
two are identical and rotate together
within the tube, being connected by
the handle (not shown). The third
is soldered to the control tube
within the body of the inhaler.
(See also Fig. 1.24).

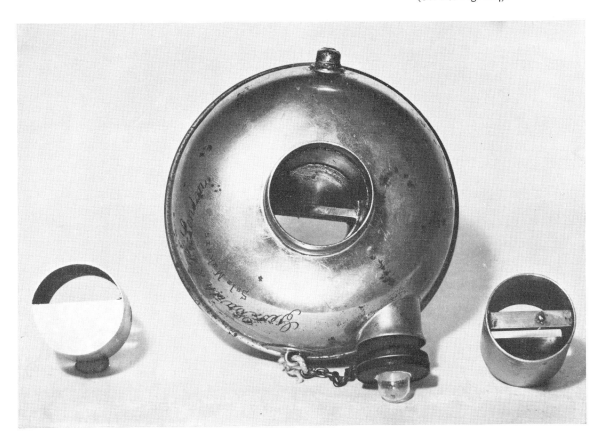

Barth & Co made the Hewitt inhaler for £3 11s 6d and appeared from their cautionary literature to have a monopoly of its construction.

Hewitt's main modifications as compared with Clover's apparatus, were:

1 increased internal calibre of the control tube and ports.

2 the central tubes, with a connecting indicator, rotated inside the ether chamber.

3 the ether filler was made wide enough and the adjustment of the ether chamber could be arranged so that refilling was possible without removing the inhaler from the face.

4 the water chamber was reduced in size and warming the apparatus prior to use was recommended.

5 the face piece was screwed to the reservoir to prevent sudden detachment (Figs. 1.22, 1.24).

ETHER APPARATUS   27

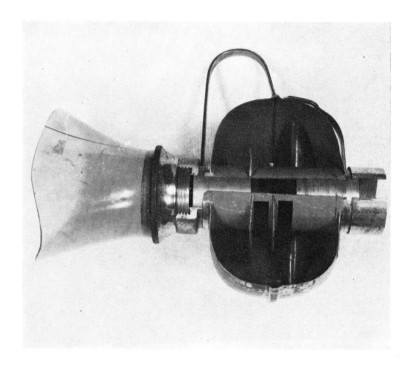

FIG. I.24. SECTIONED HEWITT
INHALER NO. O.2.16.
The segments of the inner tube are
connected by the control handle
and their ports open through the
ether chamber in the 'on' position.
The small water chamber is shown
and the celluloid mask screws into
its collar.
Geoffrey Kaye Museum, Melbourne.

CKC 19: PROBYN-WILLIAMS ETHER INHALER 1903

Robert James Probyn-Williams 1866–1952, was the first to be appointed to the post of anaesthetist to the London Hospital, though Hewitt had already become lecturer in anaesthesia at that hospital[32]. In 1901 he published *A Practical Guide to the Administration of Anaesthetics*, with a second edition in 1909 in which his inhaler was described at greater length than in the original article in the *British Medical Journal*[33, 34]. He wrote 'the body of the inhaler is pierced by two tubes, one vertical, the other horizontal. To the extremities of the vertical tube are attached the face-piece and bag respectively and through this tube the patient breathes. In the horizontal, or long axis there rotates a tube which regulates the proportion of the stream of air which is deflected into the ether chamber. The indicator is attached to the extremity of the horizontal tube and moves around part of the body of the inhaler (Figs. 1.26–1.29).

'The lumen of the vertical tube is that of an average adult trachea and as it is not contracted in any part there is no obstruction to free respiration, as there is in all forms of Clover's inhaler. The openings into the ether chamber are of the same calibre as the vertical tube.' This diameter is 22mm for both tubes, i.e. approximately the same as that for the Clover inhaler, but the absence of baffles

FIG. 1.25. CLOVER INHALER USED
FOR NITROUS OXIDE INDUCTION,
with Hewitt stopcock. Hewitt used
his own inhaler in the same manner,
attaching a gas-bag to his stopcock,
which allowed the controlled
admission of air.
From Hewitt,F.W. (1893)
Anaesthesia, p. 184

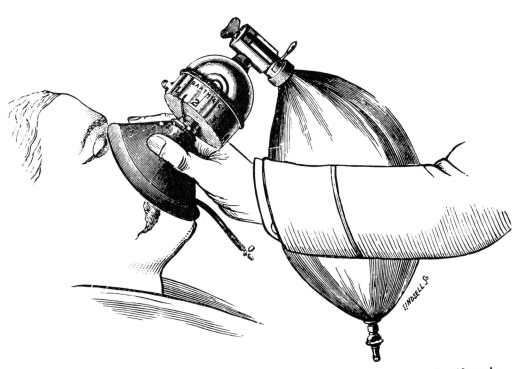

The Administration of Nitrous Oxide and Ether by means of a Clover's
Portable Ether Inhaler, a special form of Stopcock, and a detached Gas-Bag.

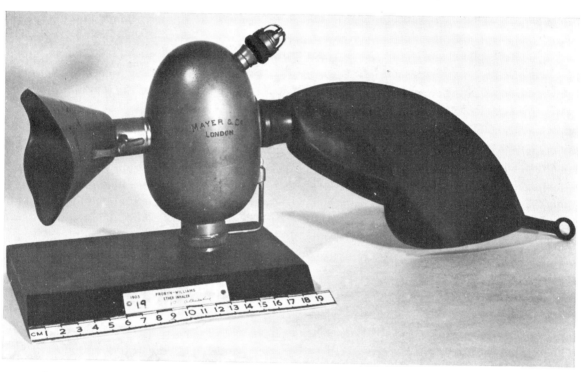

FIG. 1.26. PROBYN-WILLIAMS
ETHER INHALER, 1903.
The ovoid container was designed
to be held comfortably in the hand.
The clip which held the face piece
in one of four positions can be seen.
The bag is modern. There is no
water bath.
CKC 19

FIG. I.27. ROTATING CONTROL
TUBE OF PROBYN-WILLIAMS
INHALER.
The longitudinal baffle may be seen.
This deflects the air stream into the
ether chamber.

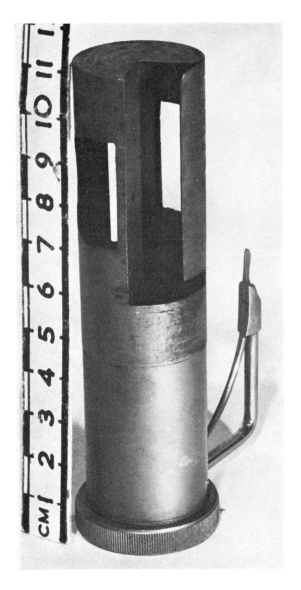

doubles the effective area. The control tube is 10cm
in length, with a diameter of 30mm.

There is no water jacket and the apparatus may be
taken apart for sterilization. The face piece is of thin
metal with a rubber air-cushion and a small metal
catch holds it very firmly in any of four positions. A
50ml ether filler is provided.

In his book (p. 106) Probyn-Williams described
how the bag angle-piece may be adapted to admit
ethyl chloride for induction. This was a method
derived from one which had first been promoted in
1902; Clover's inhaler was used, ethyl chloride
being sprayed into the bag after removal of the ether
chamber[35]. Though McCardie of Birmingham had
used ethyl chloride as a preliminary to ether in 1901,
Probyn-Williams was perhaps the first deliberately
to adapt an ether inhaler in this way[36].

The control tube of the Probyn-Williams was used
in the Bruck ether inhaler, described on p. 33.
(CKC A20) and this latter inhaler resembled the
Probyn-Williams very closely.

The Probyn-Williams inhaler presented a new
feature in design. In spite of resemblances to the
Clover and Hewitt, the introduction of the two
tubes at right angles to one another enabled the
designer to produce a tube without transverse
baffles between bag and face mask. The longer tube
is divided in its length by a baffle, but the effective
area is still about 350sq mm. Rotating the tube causes
this longitudinal strip to deflect the air stream either
directly into the bag or through the ether chamber
(see Figs. 1.28, 1.29).

FIG. I.28. DEFLECTION IN
PROBYN-WILLIAMS
rotating tube when indicator is
turned to 'full'.

FIG. I.29. WHEN INDICATOR IS
AT ZERO,
the air stream passes straight
through.
From Probyn-Williams,R.J. (1909)
*A Practical Guide to the
Administration of Anaesthetics.*
pp. 120, 121

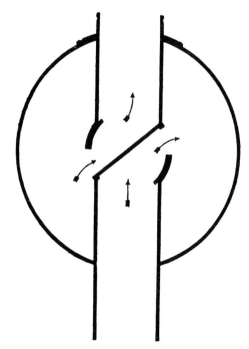

SECTION OF PROBYN-WILLIAMS' ETHER INHALER WITH
INDICATOR AT F

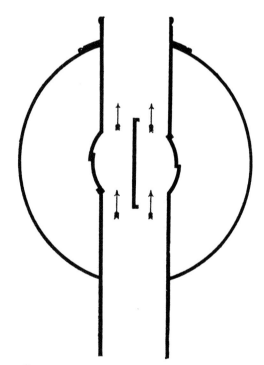

SECTION OF PROBYN-WILLIAMS' ETHER INHALER WITH
INDICATOR AT 0

FIG. 1.30. BRUCK ETHER INHALER

FIG. 1.30. BRUCK ETHER INHALER
(AFTER 1903.)
Identical with Probyn-Williams
inhaler (see p. 30) except that the
upper half of the ether chamber is
of glass. The ether measure holds
2⅓ oz (65ml). The bag is modern.
CKC A20

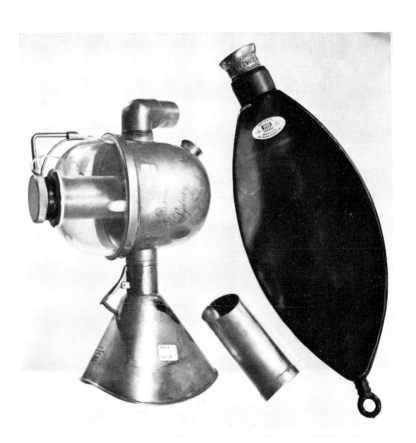

CKC A20: BRUCK MODIFIED PROBYN-WILLIAMS ETHER INHALER (after 1903)

This modified design (Figs. 1.30, 1.31) which has a control tube exactly similar to that of Probyn-Williams, (p. 31) has the name L.Bruck, Sydney, engraved, and was made by Coxeter (No.2373) with a Mayer and Meltzer bag mount. The metal cannister is, like the Probyn-Williams, ovoid in shape, and has a glass dome; a central tube, 28mm in diameter, has ports, varied by rotation, on either side, and a longitudinal baffle. The area is thus twice that of Clover's original (cf. Probyn-Williams CKC 19). A vertical cross tube, 22mm in diameter carries the face piece and bag. A metal Coxeter face piece (originally with rubber moulded pad) can be locked in one of four positions, so that the inhaler may be kept upright. An ether measure which contains 65ml ether is provided. This example possibly came from a collection made by Dr Edward Henry Embley (1861–1924) of the University of Melbourne. Dr Geoffrey Kaye mentioned such an inhaler in a letter to the President of the Association of Anaesthetists[37] in 1947; it is not certain that this is the same inhaler, since Kaye stated 'it is a modified Clover's inhaler, adapted to Hewitt's wide-bore fittings', which does not quite describe the Bruck inhaler. It is also described by Galley and King[38] as 'Embley's inhaler' and it is almost certainly one which belonged to Embley. This 'Bruck' inhaler is identical with that of Probyn-Williams, the only modification being a glass half dome to the ether chamber.

Dr Gwen Wilson of Sydney, and Dr Peter Penn, Melbourne, kindly supply the following information: 'L.Bruck, Sydney, had an instrument shop in Castlereagh Street, Sydney, for many years. He was also an instrument maker, and the modifications to the Probyn-Williams inhaler may have been carried out by him, but probably at someone else's instigation. The shop was open well into the 1930's. During the period 1900–1920 most of the anaesthetic apparatus was brought back to Sydney by returning surgeons (after FRCS, and World War I). It was usually then handed over to their favourite physician who gave the anaesthetics'[39].

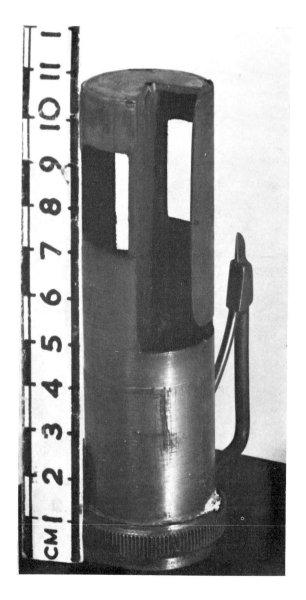

FIG. I.31. THE ROTATING TUBE
is identical with that of the Probyn-Williams inhaler.
(See Fig. I.27.)

CKC 47: OMBRÉDANNE ETHER INHALER 1908

Louis Ombrédanne, 1871–1956 (Fig. 1.32), was a Parisian surgeon with interests in paediatrics and plastic surgery[40]. He published a paper on this well-known ether inhaler in 1908[41]. In his obituary notice the inhaler is described as 'Ce bon masque exécuté primitivement avec des boites de conserves' (Figs. 1.33, 1.34). His paper was thorough and well presented and gave five propositions which he supported by diagrams of experimental apparatus. Thus his *second proposition* stated 'ether anaesthesia is unsatisfactory unless the patient breathes a mixture more or less restricted', as it was in the case of Julliard's mask with its waxed linen cover (see CKC 9, p. 254), and in the case of the Clover apparatus. Ombrédanne showed a diagram of an apparatus (Fig. 1.35) which had an opening on the inhalation tube allowing the regulated admission of fresh air. This was an improvement on his earlier designs, but he decided that it needed (1) tubes of larger section and (2) a shorter distance between the ether generator and the face mask. The latter became his *third proposition* while the *fourth proposition* stated 'the addition of fresh air is necessary . . . this proportion of fresh air is not very great.' Here he criticised Clover's inhaler (and other English apparatus) saying 'as these are not provided with means of admission of fresh air, they rapidly produce cyanosis if one does not constantly raise the mask from the face.' He also stated that 'the water chamber in the Clover apparatus is a perfectly useless element.' *The fifth proposition* is interesting as it led to the conclusion that the patient must breathe what he termed 'l'air confiné', that is, respired air from a rebreathing bag, in addition to fresh air. 'It is difficult to explain the need to breathe a relatively

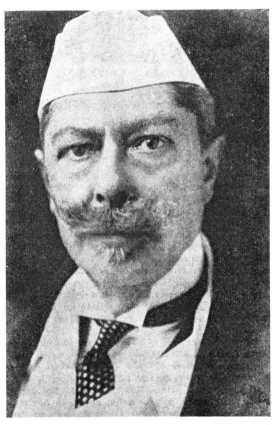

FIG. 1.32. LOUIS OMBRÉDANNE, 1871–1956, surgeon, of Paris. From *Press médicale.* (1957) **65**, 99

restricted mixture. Does the re-breathing bag permit the concentration of ether or does the inhalation of a certain amount of carbonic acid (gas) increase the narcosis? Concentration of ether vapour (as demonstrated in a special piece of apparatus which Ombrédanne designed to prevent rebreathing)* is insufficient for good anaesthesia. It is necessary therefore to admit that carbonic acid expiration

* Notes in parenthesis by K.B.T.

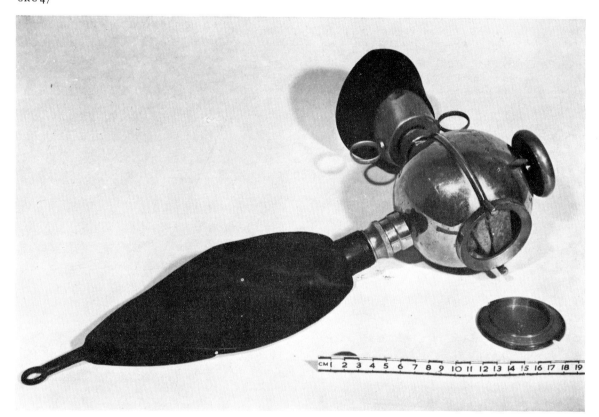

plays a useful role in anaesthesia.' Though Hewitt, for example, had mentioned the increase of carbon dioxide in a rebreathing bag[42], this observation of Ombrédanne's is probably the first to refer directly to the part played by the gas in anaesthesia.

Ombrédanne then described his own apparatus: 'a sphere filled with ether impregnated sponges is the generator (the Charles King specimen contains felt.)* It is traversed diametrically by a tube closed at one end by a sac of 'baudruche' (caecum of cow or pig)*: at the other end it opens to the external air by a stepped opening (K in Fig. 1.36 and see Fig. 1.34). On to this tube open (1) two 'chimneys' passing into the generator, (2) a tube H to the face mask and (3) a return tube J between the mask and the transverse tube (Figs. 1.36, 1.37). In the transverse tube rotates a second hollow tube, closed at N (Fig. 1.37) and pierced by windows O, O1, O2 of which O and O1 open progressively and O2 is always open. The movements of this tube are shown by an index graduated

FIG. I.34. CONTROL TUBE OF
OMBRÉDANNE INHALER.
Beside the indicator is the
'stepped' air-inlet, ('K' in fig. I.36).
The central tube rotates within a
transverse tube and the ports
engage with the 'chimneys' and
with the tube to the face mask.
(See Figs. I.36, I.37)

from 0–8. The tube is illustrated from the Charles King Collection example (Fig. I.34), where the air-inlet may be seen.

Ombrédanne then gave descriptions of the various control positions and their effect on the transit of respiration through the apparatus. For example, Fig. I.37 shows the situation when position 8 is set on the scale: 'the air window K is open to its minimum, the chimneys G are fully open: J is closed (there is therefore no direct rebreathing),★ so that there enters (1) a very small stream of fresh air (2) ether vapour saturated by passage through the sphere and derived indirectly from the closed bag'.

'Thus constructed it has given us excellent results. . . . In particular, we have sought a means of dissociating the generator from the bag (i.e. passage J)★ and we have substituted impregnated sponges for free ether.' The sponge mass is calculated to absorb 150cu cm of ether and this is sufficient for nearly all cases. Ombrédanne stated that the apparatus was not heavy, but the collection specimen weights 2 lb 2 oz (862 g). No other measurements were given, but the example from the collection shows the sphere to be 11.2mm in diameter, the chimneys open through 17mm square ports, the bag outlet is 19mm, the face piece 25mm, while the 'stepped' air-inlets have a free area of only 112sq mm (Fig. I.34). Thus although Ombrédanne was critical of Clover and Probyn-Williams for admitting no air, his own design was restricted. He was on surer ground in criticizing Clover for the internal constrictions (rétrécissements) in the tubes.

The Ombrédanne apparatus became a very popular means of 'etherization' on the continent and is thought to be still in use (Fig. I.38). It received little or no attention in England. Its popularity may have been due to this excellent explanatory paper from which a great deal may now be discovered of

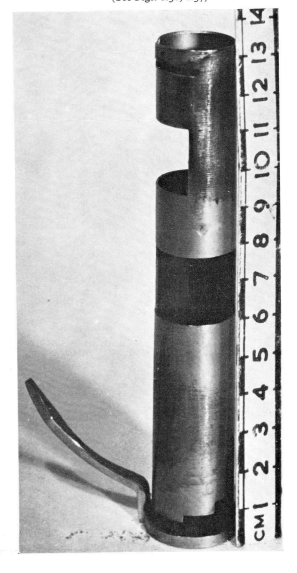

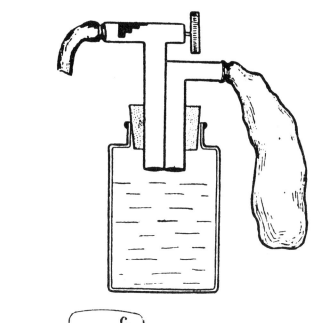

FIG. I.35. DIAGRAM FROM OMBRÉDANNE'S PAPER of 1908 illustrating his proposition 'l'anésthèsie par l'éther ne fonctionne bien que si le malade respire un milieu plus ou moins confiné.' A 'stepped' air inlet is seen on the upper tube.

FIG. I.36. SECTIONAL DIAGRAM OF OMBRÉDANNE INHALER. (See text)

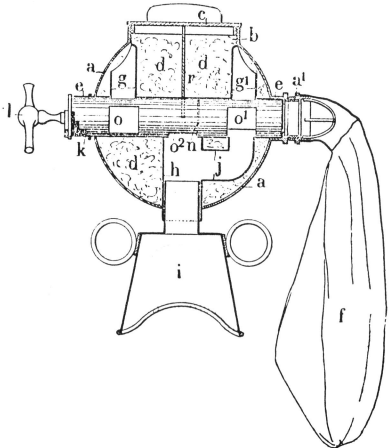

the state of respiratory physiology in relation to anaesthesia around the turn of the century.

CKC 21: BARTON ETHER INHALER 1908

George Alexander Heaton Barton MD, 1865–1924, studied at St Mary's Hospital. He became MD Brussels in 1911 and was anaesthetist to the Royal Northern Orthopaedic and Hampstead General Hospitals, London. He was killed in an accident while riding his horse in Rotten-row, Hyde Park[43], a comment upon the status of the general practitioner who practised also in a speciality! Barton wrote a number of papers, particularly on ethyl chloride[44] and in 1907 he described a sequential technique using ethyl chloride, ether and chloroform, on a Schimmelbusch mask[45].

The present apparatus was described in his book, *Backwaters of Lethe*[46] in which he made the sound observation on anaesthetic emergencies, 'It is better to do nothing well than to do the wrong thing badly'; his obituary notice states that he used somewhat elaborate methods of anaesthesia.

The apparatus consists of a cylindrical ether drum 55mm in diameter and 144mm high. The bottom is slightly bevelled 'so that when it is put down, the whole apparatus rests on the base and the edge of the face piece in fairly stable equilibrium'. About one-third of the way up the cylinder is the face piece side tube, 45mm in diameter and 22mm long, with a central constriction 23mm in diameter. The face-piece is of Roth-Dräger design, with an expiratory valve carrying a mica disc, and a rubber mask. Two versions are available. The first is represented by the Charles King Collection specimen (Fig. 1.39), in

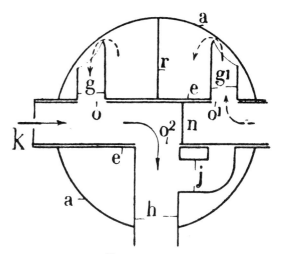

FIG 1.37. DIAGRAM OF OMBRÉDANNE INHALER when the indicator is set at 8. The air inlet K is minimal, the side tube j is closed, and the gases pass from the bag through the 'chimneys' g and g into the ether chamber and so to the face piece at h.

Figs. 1.35, 1.36, 1.37 are from Ombrédanne, L., 'Un appareil pour l'Anésthèsie par l'éther.' *Gazette des hôpitaux* (1908) 81. S1095

which ether is dropped on to lint clipped to the upper opening of the cylinder. In the second, more elaborate type (Fig. 1.40), a cap carrying an inspiratory valve fits into the top of the chamber. The latter is lined with lint and 2oz (56ml) ether is vaporized, the lining representing an evaporating surface of 20sq in. The inspiratory valve could also be placed between chamber and face piece (Fig. 1.41); in a further method of use, a rebreathing bag was

FIG.I.38. THE OMBRÉDANNE
ETHER INHALER IN USE.
Note the narrow-bore delivery tube.
From Kirschner, R. (1931)
Operative Surgery

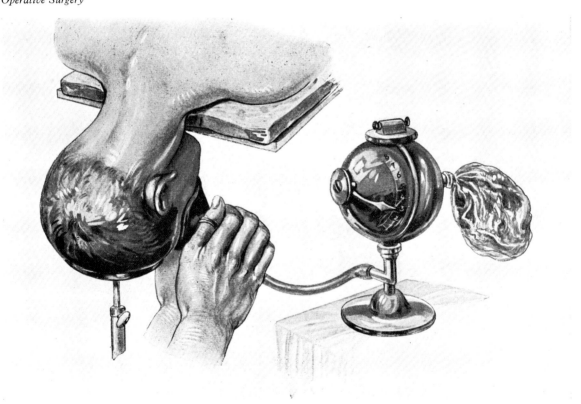

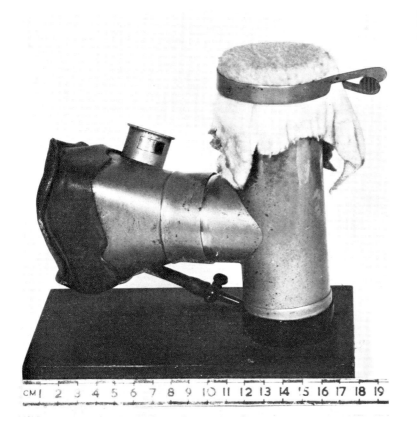

FIG. 1.39. BARTON ETHER
INHALER, 1908.
CKC 21

fitted to the top of the chamber, the inspiratory
valve being omitted and the expiratory valve closed
(Fig. 1.42). No air was admitted under these
circumstances. This somewhat primitive piece of
apparatus does not seem to have been described
elsewhere, and it is possible that only Barton himself favoured it. The provenance of the piece is unknown, but was perhaps Barton's own.

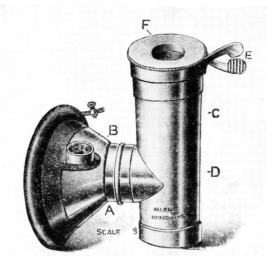

THE BARTON ETHER INHALER (ORIGINAL MODEL).

FIG. 1.40. BARTON ETHER
INHALER
showing cap with inspiratory valve.
From *Backwaters of Lethe*, (1920)
p. 17

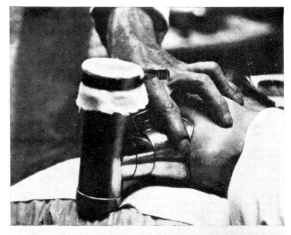

III.—IN USE AT B STRENGTH.

The inspiratory valve is now within the facepiece. The jaw is lightly
held forward by the ring finger ; the facepiece held by thumb and
forefinger ; the middle finger rests on the facial artery.

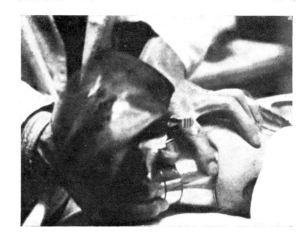

FIG. 1.42. BARTON ETHER
INHALER
fitted with rebreathing bag.
From *Backwaters of Lethe*, (1920)
Fig. IV

FIG. I.43. SILK CELLULOID
ETHER INHALER.
The oval cylinder is 6 in (15cm) in
height and is perforated at its closed
end. A sponge has been inserted, as
directed by Silk, though he
sometimes placed it in a flannel bag.
CKC 64

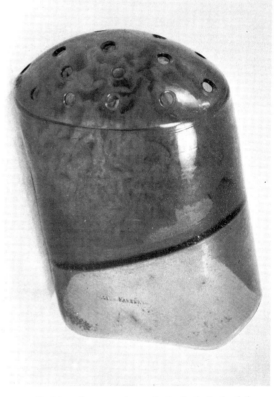

CKC 64: SILK ETHER INHALER 1894

John Frederick William Silk MD, 1848–1943, was
anaesthetist to the Great Northern Central and the
National Dental Hospitals, London, and physician
to the St Pancras Dispensary[47]. He had learned
his anaesthesia at King's College Hospital, and he
returned there in 1893, as 'anaesthetist and instructor
in anaesthetics.' He was a valuable member of the
Building Committee of the new hospital built at
Denmark Hill in 1912. Silk's contributions to
anaesthesia were many. In addition to many articles
and books [48, 49], he was a pioneer teacher and a
founder, in 1893, of the Society of Anaesthetists,
which later became the Section of Anaesthetics of
the Royal Society of Medicine.

About 1891 Silk became interested in celluloid for
face pieces, and in 1894 he described this mask
(Fig. 1.43) which is a copy of Rendle's mask, though
the latter is normally made of leather. Silk wrote 'the
value of celluloid in the construction of various
surgical appliances is gradually being recognised. For
the last two or three years I have had in constant use
a set of face-pieces and masks made of this substance. . . . The mask is made of quite stout
material . . . it is freely perforated at one end and
the other end fits lightly over the nose and mouth. A
loosely fitting flannel bag (inside the mask), serves to
protect the face and to hold in position the honey-
comb sponge upon which the anaesthetic is
poured'[50]. Silk usually employed this mask with
an alcohol/chloroform/ether mixture (see p. 211)
though for the maintenance of anaesthesia he used
ether alone.

The similarity of the design of Silk's mask to that
of Rendle is noted above. Richard Rendle produced
his in 1867, initially for the administration of
'bichloride of methylene'[51]; this substance, a mixture of chloroform and methyl alcohol, had been
introduced by Benjamin Ward Richardson in his
search for a chloroform substitute. It was much
used, especially by Spencer Wells, who first gave it
clinically in 1867, and continued with it for over
twenty years, using Junker's inhaler (see p. 73). It
may be noted that, whereas Junker's apparatus subsequently was used for chloroform, the Rendle mask
was found suitable for the administration of ether
and was popular for many years. The King Collection does not possess a specimen.

Hewitt wrote of Rendle's mask in 1901, 'with this apparatus the danger of an overdose, and of asphyxial troubles, is certainly greater than with Junker's Inhaler'[52], though Rendle himself stated that the perforations admitted just sufficient air to enable one to breath without effort [51]. In view of Hewitt's comment, it is noteworthy that he himself used Rendle's inhaler when anaesthetizing his most famous patient, King Edward VII, for the drainage of the appendicular abscess which caused the postponement of his Coronation in 1902[53].

CKC 35. 35A: PINSON ETHER 'BOMB' 1921

Kenneth Bernard Pinson of Manchester, (Fig. 1.44) now lives in Armidale, New South Wales. Such is his enthusiasm for engineering, that Dr Andrew Hunter writes that it was not safe to leave him alone with a car, so great was the itch in his fingers to take machinery apart. Out of this enthusiasm were born many pieces of anaesthetic apparatus, of which the 'bomb' is the best known; his 'Pulmo-flator', described in 1944, was an advanced closed circuit ventilator, which was never put into production. Though the 'bomb' is always known by the name of Pinson, its co-producer was a no less distinguished Manchester anaesthetist, Stanley Rawson Wilson, 1882–1927 (Fig. 1.45). In 1906, soon after he qualified, Wilson showed his aptitude for research by a statistical survey which proved the relationship between scrotal cancer and the occupation of mule-spinning[54]. It was his tragedy that he died while performing self experiments on nitrous oxide/oxygen mixtures, in which an oxygen cylinder became empty[55]. In 1927, shortly before his death, Wilson published an important paper on 'ether con-

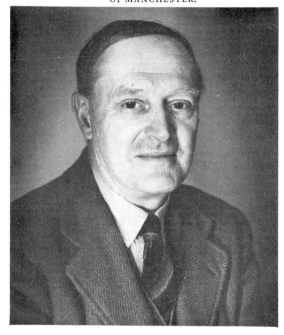

FIG. 1.44. K.B. PINSON (B. 1890) OF MANCHESTER.

vulsions', at that time a source of much worry and speculation. It would be reasonable to assume that the condition was due to the massive overdosage readily achieved with the ether 'bomb', but in the only case in which a technique is noted 'open ether' was used, and Wilson attributed the convulsions to impurities in the ether[56].

In their paper on the 'bomb' Wilson and Pinson described the advantages of warm ether, which (they wrote) diminished the loss of body heat: lessened shock: lessened secretions: is less toxic; is less irritant, less likely to cause respiratory spasm: post anaesthetic vomiting is lessened: and there is diminished risk of lung complications[57].

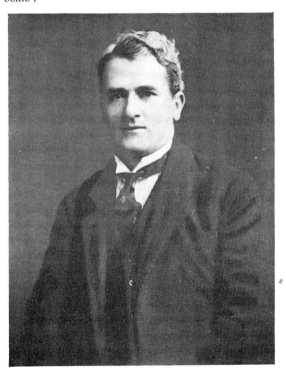

The advantages of the apparatus itself were listed as: 1, the ether is self-delivering and no bellows are required; 2, it is simple and portable in a small hand-bag; 3, there is nothing to break; 4, the delivery of the vapour can be very accurately controlled by means of a needle valve; 5, it is possible to get a stronger vapour than by other methods; 6, it is adaptable to any ordinary open mask and easily attachable to any closed nitrous oxide or ether inhaler; and 7, it affords a convenient means of anaesthetizing animals with ether if fitted either to a mask or animal box.

The strong steel vessel (Fig. 1.46) 120mm in diameter by 50 mm in height, holds 10 oz ($=$ 270ml) of ether and is tested to withstand a pressure of 250 lb sq. in. The filling aperture is closed with a screw plug and a needle-valve controls the flow of ether vapour (Fig. 1.47). Fine bore rubber tubing carries the vapour to an ordinary open ether mask. In use the vessel is plunged into hot water (no temperature given). The temperature beneath the mask is between 90° and 98°F (32°–37°C). The apparatus was made by the Condensed Gas Company, Manchester.

It is of interest to note the emphasis upon warmed ether. From the early days, attempts were made to prevent cooling by buffering with water (e.g. Snow, Clover). In the early 1900's actual warming of the ether was attempted, as by Gwathmey and Shipway. These were unsuccessful since the vapour was heated distally and arrived at the mask at virtually room temperature. The Pinson bomb is said to have delivered vapour at around body temperature, and though greater advantages were claimed for this effect than might appear justified, the inhalation of even cooler vapours possibly predisposed to the pulmonary complications of the ether era, an idea postulated by Lawson Tait as early as 1876.

Shipway[58] stated that when using an 'open ether' mask, (closely applied to the face, so that the whole of the air current in both directions, passes through the fabric), the lowering of temperature is progressive and may continue till the inhaled vapour may be 30°–40°F (17°–22°C) below the temperature of the room. Gwathmey was insistent that anaesthetics were safer at blood temperature. For example

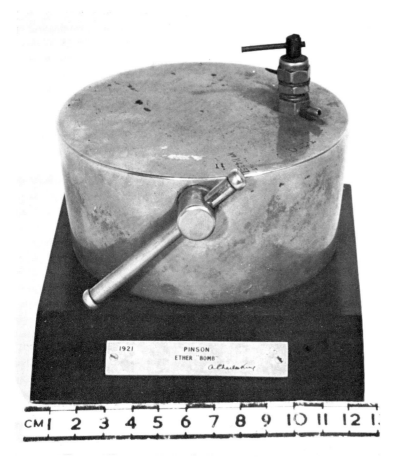

FIG. I.46. THE PINSON ETHER
BOMB, 1921.
This is an early model. Later
specimens were fitted with a
safety-valve.
CKC 35

he showed that while it took 6.57 minutes (average) to kill 16 animals with chloroform at room temperature, it took 20.35 minutes with 'warm chloroform'. Gwathmey believed that warm ether vapour is twice as safe as cold. Ross however pointed out that Gwathmey's facts were inapplicable to man, since the experimental work was done on cats and dogs who lose heat through the mouth and air-stream and that man is not a hairy animal[59]. Davis, of Johns Hopkins Hospital, found that the rectal temperature of 140 patients dropped by a mean of 1.02°F (0.5°C) using 'open ether' and in 16 patients by 0.29°F using normal vapours. These figures do not seem to be significant, but they indicate the experimental

FIG. 1.47. PINSON BOMB.
Detail of the needle valve, and
delivery tube.
From Ross & Fairlie. (1929)
Handbook of Anaesthetics, p. 144

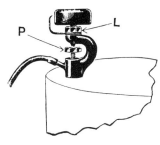

Details of the Pinson Ether Bomb. P is the packing-nut
which needs to be tightened occasionally when the action of the
valve gets loose. L is the lock-nut for re-setting the pointer.

FIG. 1.48. SIR DENIS BROWNE,
1892–1967.

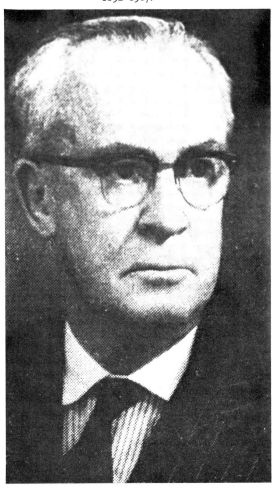

interest being shown in the subject in the first years
of the century. The matter seems finally to have been
dealt with by Seelig, who argued from theoretical
and experimental evidence that it was impossible for
a gas to retain heat during passage along 2 feet
(60cm) of tubing[60].

CKC 62: DENIS BROWNE ETHER INHALER 1928

Sir Denis Browne (Fig. 1.48) was an Australian who
came to England after the Great War. He was a
pioneer in the surgery of paediatric defects, such as
cleft palate, hypospadias and foot deformities, in
which many developments are connected with his
name. He was knighted in 1961 and died in London
in 1967[61] His own particular brand of pithy comment and mordant wit is well remembered by the
present author who worked with him in the early
years of the last war, and is well shown by the letter
to the *British Medical Journal*, quoted below, in
which he described this apparatus, the well-known
'top-hat' (Fig. 1.49). This particular example was
used by the author, working for 'D.B.' as he was
always known, at the Hospital for Sick Children,
Great Ormond Street, London. Denis Browne wrote
in 1928:

FIG. 1.49. THE DENIS BROWNE
'TOP HAT'.
The gauze pad should be an oval,
7 in (18cm) by 5 in (13cm). It is
placed over the open holder and
pushed down the outer cylinder to a
position about 1.5 in (4cm) from
the face.
CKC 62

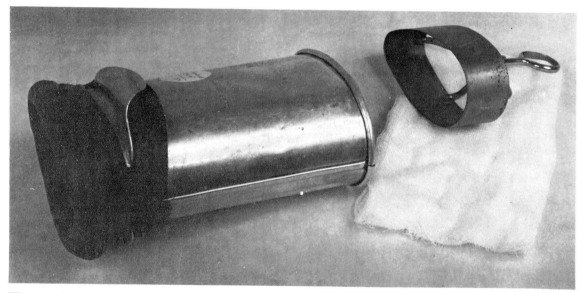

'The very interesting correspondence on the removal of tonsils and adenoids has shown that there are some who believe that this operation should be delicate and unhurried, and that the best anaesthetic for it is ether. I think that to these a description of an inhaler which has been used for three years, and in a good many thousand cases, may be of interest.

The main difficulty of giving ether is to vary the concentration of the vapour from very weak at the start to very strong when deep anaesthesia is needed. With the open method a high concentration can only be obtained by muffling the mask with towels, etc.—a crude, wasteful, and inexact proceeding. Also, the ordinary Schimmelbusch mask has the fatal defect for ether that as soon as the fluid is poured on to the convex gauze pad it runs down into its borders, leaving a dry patch through which the patient breathes.

The Clover inhaler, well used, gives a most excellent anaesthetic, but it is expensive, fragile, and difficult to clean, while its proper handling is a very rare accomplishment. Silk's inhaler has the sound principle of retaining the heavy ether vapour where it must be breathed by the patient, by means of a cylinder fitting below closely to the face. The sponge, however, when soaked with ether, is almost impermeable to air, and tends to drip from its lower surface.

My own pattern (made by Allen and Hanbury) is an aluminium "cylinder" 7 inches in height, and shaped to fit the face, with a sorbo rubber pad at the end.

The ether is held by an oval gauze pad, 7 inches by 5, and at least eight layers thick, preferably hemmed so that it can be washed and used again. This is placed on top of the cylinder, and thrust down into it, on to the bars across the lower end, by a smaller cylinder mounted on a handle. This gives a flat gauze surface, down to which all ether poured into the inhaler runs, so that the patient's breath must pass through it; while, owing to its flatness there is no tendency to dripping.

I believe this inhaler to have the following advantages.
1. It will give a very high concentration of ether with a percentage of CO_2 much as in the Clover inhaler.*
2. It is very economical, its consumption of ether being only about a third of that of the open method. In one department alone at Great Ormond Street this difference meant a saving of £50 per annum.
3. It is simple, cheap, easily cleaned between anaesthetics, and has that priceless quality for hospital equipment of surviving being dropped on a stone floor.
4. It does not cover the eyes, thus avoiding what I think to be one of the main causes of panic in children.
In using it the main points are:
1. Start the induction with a single drop of ether in the inhaler. Anyone who thinks this is too little is recommended to experiment on himself.
2. Keep the mask closely on the face, and as soon as the patient is breathing one strength of ether easily, increase it. A fairly wide experience of inducing all types of cases with ether has convinced me that the main causes of failure are starting with too strong a vapour, and taking off the mask for no particular reason except to see if the patient is still underneath it.
3. As soon as the patient is deeply anaesthetized, with dilated pupil and easy breathing, hang a weighted and hooked mouthpiece on the top of the inhaler and pump ether vapour through it. If this provokes no coughing, gag the mouth open and hang the tube in it to continue the anaesthetic, again carefully avoiding giving one breath of etherless air.

I have found this method quicker and better than inducing with ethyl chloride and changing to ether, as it avoids that "no man's land" when the patient is coming out of deep ethyl chloride into shallow ether. I think that with this method an expert operator and

anaesthetist can work at the rate of about eight cases an hour, the tonsils being dissected out and all bleeding stopped before the child leaves the table'[62].

One of his friends, writing Denis Browne's obituary notice, said: 'He made tremendous advances in a very neglected branch of surgery: evolving operations, inventing splints, gadgets and instruments each and all bearing the hall-mark of a kind of inspired simplicity.' In a lesser way the 'top-hat' also showed this quality.

CKC A2: FLAGG CAN c. 1939

Paluel Joseph Flagg, 1886–1970 (Fig. 1.50), of St Vincent's Hospital, New York, wrote a well known text-book, *The Art of Anaesthesia* in 1916, with a 6th edition in 1939. He was an important influence in American anaesthesia for his advocacy of intubation as a resuscitative method, especially in the neonate[63].

The Flagg can was first described in 1939, but Sir Robert Macintosh used it in Spain in 1938, when, under war conditions, simple portable anaesthetic apparatus was essential. Indeed, Sir Robert has told the author that here, in the Flagg can, lay the germ of the Oxford Vaporizer. The earliest design consisted merely of an ether can with perforated lid to which a tube was attached, this being connected either to a face mask, or to a pharyngeal airway (Fig. 1.51) or to an endotracheal tube. Ether could be vaporized on lint or on a sponge within the can. Later modifications included the use of a side draw tube, the top of the can being covered by gauze on to which ether was dropped as in the present example.

* One must doubt the truth of this statement, remembering the completely closed nature of the Clover inhaler. K.B.T.

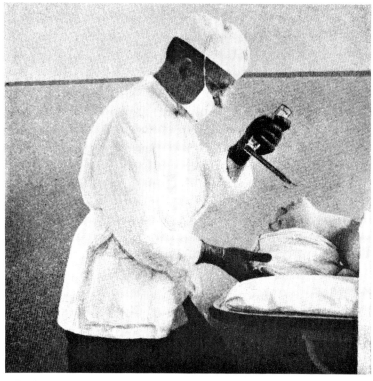

FIG. I.50. PALUEL JOSEPH
FLAGG, M.D.
Demonstrating intubation, using
the technique of Chevalier Jackson.
From Flagg, Paluel, (1939). *The Art
of Anaesthesia*, p. 164.

In the Western Desert in 1940, Dr Geoffrey Kaye, adviser in anaesthesia to the Australian Imperial Force, made up Flagg cans from discarded tins. He writes 'in field ambulances, even the simple ether vaporiser was an undue burden, so resort was made to a modified Flagg can. Such cans were made up at Al-Qantara from Army ration cream-tins'[64, 65].

The present example is rather more sophisticated. The specially made can is $3\frac{1}{2}$in (90mm) in diameter and depth, and has a circular spring holding the vaporizing gauze. An outlet tube $\frac{1}{2}$ in (12.5mm) in diameter, issues from the tin $\frac{3}{4}$ in (22mm) from the top for connection by rubber tube to a pharyngeal or endotracheal tube (Fig. 1.52). The Flagg can provided a simple, easily made emergency type of ether vaporiser. Cooling does not seem to have been a problem, possibly because of its use in warm climates, vaporization also being aided in the later models, by dripping the ether on to the gauze cover. Earlier models were less safe in that tilting the can could allow liquid ether to run into the outlet tube.

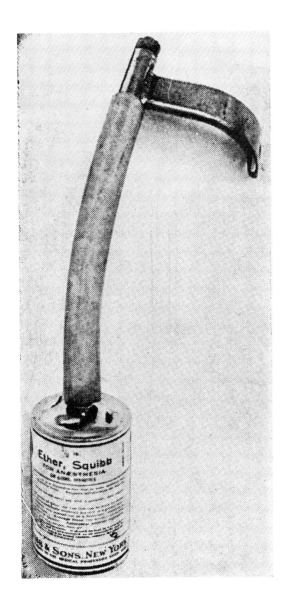

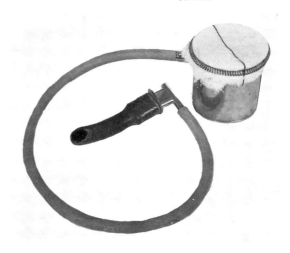

FIG. 1.51. FLAGG CAN
as described by Flagg himself.
From *The Art of Anaesthesia*, (1939)
p. 148

FIG. 1.52. FLAGG CAN
with Phillip's airway.
CKC A2

REFERENCES

1 YOUNG H.H. (1897) Long, the discoverer of anaesthesia. *Johns Hopkins Hosp. Bull.* **8**, 182.

2 BIGELOW H.J. (1846) Insensibility during operations produced by inhalation. *Boston med. and surg. J.* **xxv**, 312.

3 DUNCUM B. (1947) *Development of Inhalation Anaesthesia.* London: Oxford University Press, p. 133.

4 SNOW J. (1847) *On the Inhalation of the Vapour of Ether in surgical operations.* London: Churchill, pp. 16, 17.

5 MORTON W.T.G. (1847) Letter from Dr Morton. *Lancet,* **ii**, 80.

6 HAYWARD J.W. (1871) On Ether and chloroform as anaesthetics. *Med. Times.* **ii**, 603.

7 HEWITT F.W. (1893) *Anaesthetics and their Administration.* London: Griffin, p. 184.

8 ORMSBY L.H. (1877) A new ether inhaler. *Lancet.* **i**. 218.

9 HEWITT F.W. (1893) *op. cit.* p. 151.

10 EPSTEIN H.G., MACINTOSH R.R., & MENDELSOHN K., (1941) The Oxford vaporizer no. 1. *Lancet,* **ii**, 62–64.

11 GWATHMEY J.T. (1914) *Anesthesia.* New York: Appleton, p. 13.

12 DUNCUM B. (1947) *op. cit.* Ch. III.

13 THOMAS K.B. (1968) Centenary of a benefactor. *Anaesthesia,* **23**, 676.

14 Obituary notice: John Snow, M.D. (1858). *Med. Times and Gazette,* n.s. **16**, 633.

15 SNOW J. (1858) *On Chloroform.* London: Churchill. Biography by B.W.Richardson, pp. i–xliv.

16 SNOW J. (1847) *op. cit.* pp. 16, *et seq.*

17 SNOW J (1847) *op. cit.* p. 20.

18 SNOW J. (1847) *op. cit.* p. 23.

19 Obituary notices: (1882) Joseph Thomas Clover. *Brit. med. J.* **ii**, 656; and *Lancet,* **ii**, 597.

20 CLOVER J.T. (1877) Portable regulating ether inhaler. *Brit. med. J.* **i**, 69–70.

21 PROBYN-WILLIAMS R.J. (1909) *Practical Guide to the Administration of Anaesthetics.* London: Longmans, Green, 2nd edn, pp. 116, 117.

22 GALLEY A.H., & KING, A. CHARLES (1948) Modifications of the Clover's ether inhaler. *Anaesthesia,* **3**, 147.

23 Obituary notice: T.Wilson-Smith (1955) *Brit. med. J.* **ii**, 497.

24 GALLEY A.H. & KING, A. CHARLES. (1948) *op. cit.* p. 148.

25 WILSON-SMITH T. (1898) Improved ether inhaler. *Lancet,* **i**, 1005.

26 WILSON-SMITH T. (1899) Inhaler (Clover's) modified. *Medical Annual.* Bristol: J.Wright, p. 647.

27 WILSON-SMITH T. (1899) *ibid.,* p. 648.

28 GALLEY A.H. & KING, A. CHARLES (1948) *op. cit.* p. 149.

29 Obituary notice: Sir Frederick Hewitt (1916) *Brit. med. J.* **i**, 113.

30 HEWITT F.W. (1901) *Anaesthetics.* London: Griffin, 2nd ed, p. 277.

31 GARDNER H. BELLAMY (1916) *A Manual of Surgical Anaesthesia.* Toronto: Macmillan, 2nd edn, p. 127.

32 Obituary notices: R.J.Probyn-Williams (1953) *Brit. med. J.* **i**, 47; *Anaesthesia,* **8**, 129.

33 PROBYN-WILLIAMS R.J. (1909) *op. cit.* p. 119.

34 PROBYN-WILLIAMS R.J. (1903) A wide-bore regulating ether inhaler. *Brit. med. J.* **ii**, 593.

35 DUNCUM B. (1947) *op. cit.* p. 509

36 McCARDIE W.J. (1901) A few cases of ethyl chloride narcosis. *Lancet.* **i**, 698.

37 KAYE G. (1947) Letter to President (of the Association of Anaesthetists). *Anaesthesia,* **2**, 82.

38 GALLEY A.H., & KING, A. CHARLES. (1948) *op. cit.* p. 150.

39 Dr GWEN WILSON, SYDNEY. *Personal Communication.* 1972.

40 Obituary notice: Louis Ombrédanne. (1957) *Presse Médicale,* **65**, 99 (16 Jan).

41 OMBRÉDANNE L. (1908). Un Appareil pour l'anesthésie par l'éther. *Gaz. des. Hôpitaux,* **81**, S1095.

42 HEWITT F.W. (1901). *op. cit.* p. 49.

43 Obituary notices: G.A.H. Barton (1924). *Lancet,* **i**, 155 and *Brit. med. J.* **i**, 135.

44 BARTON, G.A.H. (1905). *A Guide to the Administration of Ethyl Chloride.* London: Lewis.

45 BARTON G.A.H. (1907). The CE—Ethyl Chloride-Chloroform Sequence. *Practitioner*, **79**, ii, 791.

46 BARTON G.A.H. (1920). *Backwaters of Lethe (some anaesthetic notions)*. London: Lewis, pp. 17–24.

47 Obituary notice: (1943). John Frederick William Silk. *Brit. med. J.* **ii**, 731.

48 SILK, J.F.W. (1888). *A Manual of Nitrous Oxide Anaesthesia*. London: Churchill, pp. 120.

49 SILK J.F.W. (1914). *Modern Anaesthetics*. London: Arnold, pp. 200.

50 SILK J.F.W. (1894). Celluloid Face-Pieces and Masks for the Administration of Anaesthetics. *Lancet*, **i**, 98.

51 RENDLE R. (1869). . . . On a new method of producing rapid anaesthesia with bichloride of methylene. *Brit. med. J.* **ii**, 412.

52 HEWITT F.W. (1901). *op. cit.* p. 399.

53 *Hewitt's Diary*. Personal communication from Professor J.D.Robertson, Edinburgh, 1974.

54 [WILSON S.R.] (1927). Scrotal cancer in Cotton Mule-Spinners. *Brit. Med. J.* **ii**, 993. *Post. obit. annotation.*

55 Obituary notices: (1927). S.R.Wilson. *Brit. med. J.* **ii**, 570. *Brit. J. Anaesth.* **5**, 67–80.

56 WILSON S.R. (1927). 'Ether' Convulsions. *Lancet*, **i**, 1117.

57 WILSON S.R. & PINSON K.B. (1921). A Warm Ether Bomb. *Lancet*, **i**, 336.

58 SHIPWAY F. (1916). The Advantages of Warm Anaesthetic Vapours . . . *Lancet*, **i**, 70.

59 ROSS STUART (1919). *Handbook of Anaesthetics*. Edinburgh: Livingstone. p. 90.

60 SEELIG M.G. (1911). The Fallacy of Warmed Ether Vapour. *Interstate Med. J.* **18**, 927.

61 Obituary notices: (1967). Sir Denis Browne. *Brit. med. J.* **i**, 178, 508. *Lancet*, **i**, 166.

62 BROWNE D. (1928). Anaesthesia for Tonsillectomy and Removal of Adenoids. *Brit. med. J.* **ii**, 632.

63 Obituary notice: (1970). Paluel J.Flagg. *American Society of Anesthesiologists Newsletter.* **34**, 3. p. 6.

64 KAYE GEOFFREY. *Personal communication*, 1972.

65 KAYE GEOFFREY (1942). *Australian Army Manual of Anaesthetic Apparatus.* p. 49.

Section II
The Chloroform Series

ILLUSTRATIONS

Frontispiece Dr M.H.Armstrong–
Davison, first Curator of the Charles
King Collection. (Photograph kindly
supplied by Mrs Armstrong–
Davison, through Dr John
Inkster.)

2.1 Sir James Young Simpson
1811–1870 (from a photograph in
The Library, Royal Society of
Medicine, Courtesy of the
Librarian).

2.2 James Matthews Duncan 1826–
1890.

2.3. George Keith (courtesy of Mrs
Chapman of Deal)

2.4 Chloroform Committees and
Commissions (Courtesy of the
Honorary Editors, *Proceedings of
the Royal Society of Medicine*.)

2.5 Alfred Coleman 1828–1902
(from Duncum.B. (1947)
*Development of Inhalation
Anaesthesia*. Courtesy of the
Wellcome Trustees.

2.6 Goodman Levy's tracing of the
effect of adrenalin on the lightly
chloroformed cat. (Courtesy of
the Editor, *Journal of Physiology*.)

2.7 Edward William Murphy 1802–
1877 (from Herbert,B.T. and
Edwards,E. (1867) *Photographs of
eminent medical men*. London:
Churchill, vol. 1, p. 69. Courtesy
of The Wellcome Trustees).

2.8 Murphy chloroform inhaler
1850. CKC 3.

2.9 Murphy chloroform inhaler
(from Murphy,E. (1862) *Lectures
on the Principles and Practice of
Midwifery*. London: Walton and
Maberly, 2nd ed., p. 576.
Author's copy).

2.10 Title page of Murphy,E.W.
(1855) *Chloroform; its properties
and safety in Childbirth*. London:
Walton and Maberly. (Courtesy
of the Librarian, Royal Society of
Medicine.)

2.11 Arthur Ernest Sansom 1838–
1907 (Courtesy of the Editor,
Lancet).

2.12 Title page of Sansom (1865)
on *Chloroform* (Author's copy.)

2.13 Sansom chloroform inhaler
1880. CKC 11.

2.14 Sansom chloroform inhaler
(from Duncum,B. (1947)
*Development of Inhalation
Anaesthesia*, p. 238. Courtesy of
the Wellcome Trustees).

2.15 Sansom chloroform inhaler
(from Sansom,A.E. (1865)
*Chloroform. Its Action and
Administration*. London:
Churchill. p. 127).

2.16 Junker chloroform inhaler
1867 (from *Medical Times and
Gazette*, 1867, **ii**, 590).

2.17 Junker bottle in its early
(unsafe) state. CKC A17.

2.18 Dudley Buxton's modification
of Junker inhaler. CKC 63.

2.19 Modifications of the Junker
bottle.

2.20 Hewitt's modification of
Junker bottle, *c.* 1890 (from
Hewitt,F. (1901) *Anaesthetics and
their Administration*. London:
Macmillan, 2nd ed, p. 316.
Author's copy).

2.21 Hewitt's Junker bottle, as
worn (from Hewitt,F. (1901).,
ibid.).

2.22 Further modification by
Hewitt of Junker inhaler (from
Hewitt,F. (1893) *Anaesthetics and
their Administration*. London:
Griffin, p. 195. Author's copy).

2.23 Carter–Braine's modification
of Junker inhaler (from Carter–
Braine (1892) A Safety Junker
inhaler. *Brit. med. J.*, **i**, 1364.
Courtesy of the Editor).

2.24 Mouth tube for use with
Junker inhaler (from Hewitt,F.
(1893), *op. cit.*, p. 199).

2.25 Mason gag with cloroform
tube, for use with Junker inhaler
(from Hewitt,F. (1893), *op. cit.*,
p. 200).

2.26 Friedrich Trendelenburg
1844–1924.

2.27 Hahn tracheotomy tube
1871. CKC 6.

2.28 Trendelenburg cone 1869.

2.29 Hahn sponge and
Trendelenburg balloon cuffs
(from Probyn-Williams,R.J.
(1909) *Practical Guide for the
Administration of Anaesthetics*.
London: Longmans, Green.
2nd ed., p. 156. Author's
copy).

2.30 Trendelenburg tampon
cannula (from Kirschner,M.
(1931) *Operative Surgery*, trans.
Ravdin. Philadelphia:
Lippincott, p. 156. Courtesy of
the publishers).

2.31 Hahn sponge tracheotomy
tube (from Kirschner,M. (1931),
ibid. Courtesy of the publishers).

2.32 Augustus Vernon Harcourt,
F.R.S. 1834–1919 (from *Proc.
Roy. Soc. Series A*. 1920. **97**, vii.
Courtesy of the Editor).

2.33 Vernon Harcourt chloroform
inhaler 1903. CKC 20.

2.34 Double-necked chloroform
bottle: Vernon Harcourt inhaler
(from Buxton,D.W. (1914)
*Anaesthetics, their Uses and
Administration*. London: Lewis,
5th ed., p. 244).

2.35 Mixture control of the
Vernon Harcourt inhaler.

2.36 Unidirectional valve of Vernon Harcourt inhaler.

2.37 Vernon Harcourt chloroform inhaler in use (from Buxton,D.W. (1914), *op. cit.* pl. v).

2.38 Vernon Harcourt inhaler for hospital use (from Buxton,D.W. 1914), *ibid.*, p. 244).

2.39 Augustus Desiré Waller, F.R.S. 1856–1922, with his bulldog, Jimmie (from Burch and de Pasquale (1964) *A History of Electrocardiography*. Chicago: Year Book Medical Pub. Courtesy of the publishers).

2.40 Effects of ether and chloroform on the electrical state of a nerve (from Waller,A.D. (1910) *Physiology, the Servant of Medicine*. London: Univ. of London Pr., p. 32. Courtesy of the publishers. Author's copy).

2.41 Waller chloroform balance (Courtesy of Penlon Ltd., Abingdon).

2.42 Controls of Waller balance (Courtesy of Penlon Ltd., Abingdon).

2.43 Diagram of Waller balance (from Waller,A.D. (1910), *op. cit.* p. 109).

2.44 Waller chloroform balance revisited. An electronic version made by Drs J.W.C. and E.Fox, and presented to the Charles King Collection. CKC 61

2.45 Hirsch chloroform inhaler (from *Lancet*, 1916, **i**, 730. Courtesy of the Editor).

2.46 Hirsch percentage chloroform inhaler 1916. CKC 27.

2.47 Sudeck chloroform inhaler, *c.* 1900. CKC 70.

2.48 Sudeck inhaler, interior of face piece to show valves.

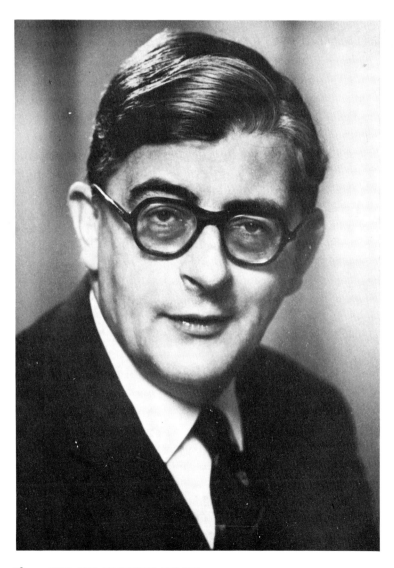

DR M.H. ARMSTRONG DAVISON,
1911–1970.
Anaesthetist and historian, he was
the first Curator of the Charles
King Collection, and a keen
protagonist of chloroform
anaesthesia over many years.

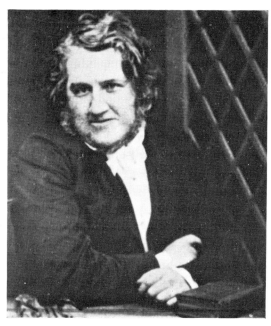

FIG. 2.1. SIR JAMES YOUNG
SIMPSON, 1811–1870,
pioneer of ether anaesthesia in
midwifery. First experiment with
chloroform, 4 November 1847. His
first paper was read on 10 November
and within a few weeks he himself
had given chloroform to fifty
Edinburgh ladies in childbirth.

INTRODUCTION: *CHLOROFORM AND CONTROVERSY*

On 19 January 1847, two months after its first use in Britain, James Young Simpson 1811–1870 (Fig. 2.1) Professor of Obstetrics at Edinburgh, was the first to use *ether* in midwifery. As a humane physician and a brilliant exponent of new ideas Simpson was quick to seize upon the principle, and was full of enthusiasm for the drug. At first he employed ether anaesthesia for patients requiring forceps or operative deliveries, but soon was using it in normal deliveries. However, he found disadvantages in 'the disagreeable and very persistent smell, its occasional tendency to irritation of the bronchi during its first inspirations, and the large quantity occasionally required to be used . . .' 'Latterly' he wrote 'I have tried upon myself and others the inhalation of different other volatile fluids . . .'[1] Thus he came upon chloroform; the story is well known of his experiment, after supper, upon himself and his junior colleagues, Doctors Matthews Duncan (Fig. 2.2) and George Keith (Fig. 2.3) at his house in Queen Street. The surgeon, Professor James Miller, for whom Simpson anaesthetised, was a near neighbour; knowing of the experiments he made a habit of calling at number 52 in the morning to see that all was well after the nocturnal inhalations. Miller has recorded that on the famous occasion Simpson woke up first, but Duncan continued to snore under the table and Keith was kicking violently, while Mrs Simpson and her nieces were in a state of considerable alarm[2]. The date was 4 November 1847. The first obstetric delivery under chloroform took place next day: five days later Simpson reported to the Medico-Chirurgical Society of Edinburgh and on 15 November his first pamphlet was published, a preliminary notice having already appeared on the 12th[3]. Thus chloroform anaesthesia was born, experimented on and publicised within the narrow space of eleven days. Those who opposed him—and there were many—were attacked and counter-attacked by Simpson in the same vigorous and immediate fashion, and his pamphlet replying to the religious objectors appeared early in 1848[4].

Simpson was not the first to use chloroform as an anaesthetic. The substance called chloric ether, which was a solution of chloroform in alcohol, had been in use as an antispasmodic in asthma for some years. In 1847, Jacob Bell had used it as an anaesthetic for dental cases at the Middlesex Hospital[5] and in November William Lawrence was 'in the habit of directing its administration' at St Bartholomew's Hospital[6].

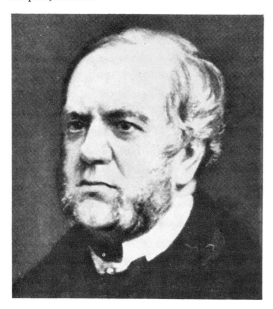

the inherent properties of the drug itself. Within three months of its discovery, Hannah Greener had died from its use and though Simpson himself tended to play down the action of the drug as the cause of death, others were more realistic and, fatalities continuing, the remainder of the nineteenth century was taken up with Committees and Commissions which failed to solve the problems (see Fig. 2.4). In fact, in spite of all their recommendations and findings, anaesthetists continued to use chloroform for its convenience and ease of administration. John Snow had posed the question in 1858, and had given some part of the answer. Snow had quoted the experiments of Dr R.M.Glover of Newcastle; as early as 1842, Glover had shown that the drug induced irritability of the heart in frogs, and Snow himself showed that the motion of the frog's heart 'can be arrested by an amount of chloroform somewhat greater than suffices to suspend the respiration'

Chloroform itself had been discovered independently in 1831 by Soubeiran in France and by Samuel Guthrie of New York. In 1832, Leibig analysed a sample which he prepared by the same method of distilling alcohol with chloride of lime. His analysis was erroneous. The French chemist Dumas named the substance chloroform in 1834, and subsequently produced a correct analysis[7]. In discussion with Simpson, David Waldie, chemist, of Liverpool, suggested a trial of chloroform and may have mentioned its properties. There were later recriminations over this dialogue; Waldie accused Simpson of failure to acknowledge his claims, though there can be no doubt that Simpson's was the genius behind its introduction into anaesthesia.

Controversy in the case of chloroform, however, arose less from clashes of personalities, than from

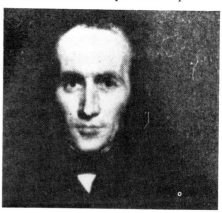

FIG. 2.3. GEORGE KEITH c. 1870.
Shared the original chloroform
experiment with Simpson and
Duncan, after dinner, 4 November
1847.

CHLOROFORM COMMITTEES AND COMMISSIONS

1864	Royal Medico-Chirurgical Society – mixtures.
1877	The Glasgow Committee– ethidene.
1888	First Hyderabad Commission – respiration, not heart.
1889	Second Hyderabad Commission – asphyxia, not vagus or heart.
1891	B.M.A. Anaesthetics Committee – $CHCL_3$ high mortality.
1893	Lancet questionnaire – Simpson's handkerchief common.
1901	B.M.A. Special Chloroform Committee – 2% Chloroform.
1912	A.M.A. Committee on Anaesthesia – Ban Chloroform.

FIG. 2.4. THE CHLOROFORM COMMISSIONS AND COMMITTEES of forty-eight years, with their recommendations. [18]

[8]. Snow, as the protagonist of the use of a controlled percentage of chloroform vapour in the inspired mixture, based his argument on the study of some fifty fatal cases, which he discussed in his great book, *On Chloroform*. He argued from his previous experiments 'that chloroform vapour has the effect of suddenly arresting the action of the heart when it is mixed with the respired air to the extent of eight or ten per cent. or upwards: and we must therefore conclude that in the fatal cases of its inhalation, the air the patients were breathing just before the accidents occurred contained this amount of vapour'[9]. 'The first rule, therefore, in giving chloroform is to take care that the vapour is so far diluted that it cannot cause sudden death without timely warning: and the next rule is to watch the symptoms as they arise'[10]. Thus Snow realized the need for careful observation of the pulse, as well as the respiration, but was in error in assuming that sudden overdosage was responsible for the deaths. The Scottish school maintained that it was never necessary to watch the pulse, the respiration always failing first. Snow accepted this in some instances, but in discussing artificial respiration, he wrote 'The fact of the breathing continuing after the action of the heart has ceased, in some of the fatal cases, shows that the heart may be so paralysed as not to be readily restored by the breathing . . .'[11] It is of interest that Snow described a case of collapse revived by

Mr Fergusson who 'applied his mouth to that of the patient and with a very strong expiration, inflated her lungs. . . . I immediately heard the heart's action recommence with very rapid and feeble strokes . . . natural breathing and pulse were soon re-established.' Yet on the same page, Snow wrote 'The most ready and effectual mode of performing artificial respiration is undoubtedly the postural method introduced by Dr Marshall Hall . . .'[12], a strange failure to recognize an important principle.

Snow's insistence upon a low, measured percentage of chloroform led, in England, to the development of inhalers and apparatus in a manner which was not followed elsewhere, though in France in particular there were those who described many ingenious pieces of apparatus, such as Duroy's anaesthesiometer, 1857; this complicated machine was stated to have required 25 minutes for induction of anaesthesia[13]. Snow himself described the idea of a bag or balloon containing 4 per cent of chloroform vapour in air, 'but I have not often resorted to this plan, on account of its being somewhat troublesome'[14]. It was left to Joseph Thomas Clover, 1825–1882, to make use of this idea in his famous chloroform bag, used with less trouble by slinging it over the shoulder (Fig. 1.10).

As the century advanced, new ideas appeared. In 1869 the great German surgeon, Friedrich Trendelenburg, 1844–1924, suggested the use of a

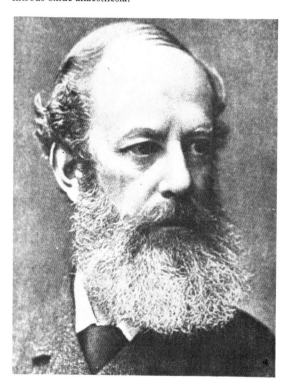

cuffed tracheotomy tube through which chloroform
was inhaled, for operations on larynx and pharynx:
the Hahn/Trendelenburg apparatus (CKC 6. Fig.
2.27) demonstrates this concept, and was described
in detail by Ferdinand Ethelbert Junker in 1872[15]
(see p. 83). Junker himself in 1867 invented a famous
and successful apparatus, used in various forms for
many years, (CKC 17/63/A17, Fig. 2.17) and making
use of a new idea, the 'blow-over' principle being substituted for the 'draw-over.' While this was probably
the first successful use of this principle, it had been
suggested a few years before by Alfred Coleman,

1828–1902 (Fig. 2.5), the London dental surgeon
whose important contributions to dental anaesthesia
gave so much impetus to the development of that
branch of the subject.

To this period also belongs the development of
the wire frame mask, originated in 1862 by the
Liverpool obstetrician Thomas Skinner, eponym-
ically developed as the Schimmelbusch mask in
1890, (see p. 250 and Figs. 7.3, 7.4), and used for
ether as well as chloroform.

In the meantime, the Scottish school had continued Simpson's practice of 'open' chloroform,
under the influence of the surgeons, James Syme,
1799–1870, and Joseph Lister, 1827–1912. It was
their insistence that death was due primarily to
respiratory failure resulting from overdose, and not
to cardiac failure, which led Syme's pupil, Edward
Lawrie, 1846–1915[16, 17], on his egotistical cam-
paign, and this in turn resulted in the Hyderabad
Commissions of 1888 and 1889[18].

Lister conducted experimental work which tended to show that the strength of chloroform under
the mask was not more than 4.5 per cent. In 1871 he
wrote 'a folded towel on which the anaesthetic liquid
is poured, unmeasured and unstinted, is still the only
apparatus employed: preliminary examination of the
heart is never thought of and . . . the pulse is
entirely disregarded: but vigilant attention is kept
upon the respiration. . . .' He added that 'the
appointment of a special chloroform giver to a
hospital is entirely unnecessary'[19].

The insistence that the heart was unimportant as
compared with the respiration was the main source
of contention until well into the present century; it
resulted in violent antagonism between the English
and Scottish schools. Snow and his followers
believed that low percentages of chloroform (up to
4 per cent) in air should be given, and though Syme

and Lister agreed that high percentages caused cardiac failure, they would not admit that chloroform deaths occurred if the respiration were watched. Yet the journals weekly were reporting fatalities following induction with chloroform, and the setting up of the Medico-Chirurgical Society Chloroform Committee 1864, and the Glasgow Committee of 1877, was followed by the two Hyderabad Commissions and the British Medical Association Committees of 1891 and 1901 (Fig. 2.4). Thus at about ten year intervals over a period of nearly forty years, the best brains of the profession failed to find satisfactory answers. Many factors militated against them, not the least important of which was the failure to understand species differences. Wood and Hare pointed out in 1890 that the Indian pariah dog (as used in Hyderabad) is a different animal from its European counterpart, adding that 'a well-established clinical fact cannot be disproved by any amount of experiments on animals'[20]. In due course, Goodman Levy was to make his important contribution, using cats, whose cardiac neuromuscular mechanism is now known to be far more susceptible to light chloroform anaesthesia than is that of the dog.

Following the Hyderabad Commissions, a great deal of physiological investigation was concentrated upon the effects of chloroform. Thus Gaskell and Shore of Cambridge, in 1893, after a brilliant series of cross-circulation experiments, found, *inter alia*, a direct action of chloroform upon the heart[21]. In 1887 J.A.McWilliam of Aberdeen had been the first to demonstrate ventricular fibrillation, showing also that certain poisons could produce this phenomenon. Among the twenty-four conclusions at which McWilliam arrived were the following:

'1. During chloroform anaesthesia the blood pressure is lowered and the heart is weakened.

2. Dilatation of the heart occurs to an appreciable extent, even when chloroform is administered gently, mixed with abundance of air (under four per cent chloroform vapour).

11. The depressing influence of chloroform on the heart . . . is not exerted through the vagus nerves, but is a direct effect of the drug upon the cardiac mechanism'[22].

Even then the unbelievers were not converted, but these conclusions, with other similar findings and arguments, led to the setting up of the 1901 Chloroform Committee of the British Medical Association under the chairmanship of Professor Augustus D.Waller (Fig. 2.39) of the University of London (see p. 89); this Committee was responsible for the suggestion that chloroform should not be administered in higher concentrations than two per cent. As a result a number of forms of percentage apparatus were produced, notably those of Waller himself (CKC 61, Fig. 2.41) Vernon Harcourt (CKC 20, Fig. 2.33) Goodman Levy [23], B.J. Collingwood[24], and others.

In 1911 came the work of Goodman Levy who had been resident anaesthetist at Guy's Hospital; in a paper read to the Physiological Society[25] Levy described 'a hitherto unrecognised form of sudden cardiac failure which occurred in cats under chloroform.' Acting on a suggestion made by Professor Arthur Cushney, then Professor of Pharmacology in the University of London, Levy looked for ventricular fibrillation. In three cases, he found the ventricules dilated and fibrillating, with complete absence of pulsation. At the same time he showed that the same form of death could be produced by injecting small doses of adrenalin into the vein of a lightly chloroformed cat. Levy's tracing (Fig. 2.6) shows sudden heart failure in a tracheotomized chloroformed cat (1.5 per cent chloroform in air) occurring 55 seconds after induction, respiration

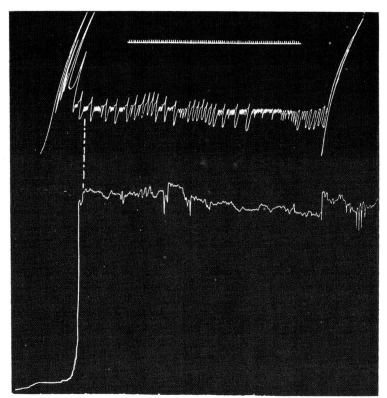

ceasing 18 seconds later. Levy also postulated the similar effect of endogenous adrenalin (see p. 89).

Though this was in fact the final blow to chloroform, anaesthetists were slow to recognize that this was so, and apparatuses in the Charles King Collection of as late a date as 1930, show the addition of a chloroform bottle as standard (see i. *Shipway*. Warm ether and chloroform apparatus, 1916 (CKC 25, p. 182, Fig. 4.7). ii. *Boyle*, gas-oxygen-ether-chloroform apparatus, 1930. (CKC 41, p. 146, Fig. 3.50)). In 1930 also, Rood and Webber of University College Hospital were, surprisingly, to write regarding circulatory failure—'the injection of adrenalin during chloroform anaesthesia, especially if the anaesthetic is light, is said to have a certain risk, but we have not seen a case where harm has resulted. . . .'[26] This was 18 years after Goodman Levy!

Latterly it has been suggested that in light chloroform anaesthesia, cardiac arrest may occur in systole as well as following ventricular fibrilla-tion[27]. The continuing enthusiasm for chloroform displayed by Dr M.H.Armstrong Davison (frontispiece) has already been noticed, and Ralph Waters in 1951 surveyed its use as though it were a newly discovered drug. That interest in chloroform continues is shown by the recent work of Oduntan, (*Anaesthesia*, (1968), **23**, 552), suggesting that the drug could be administered with a degree of safety equal to that of halothane, and advocating its use in underdeveloped countries.

CKC 3: MURPHY CHLOROFORM INHALER *c.* 1850

Edward William Murphy, M.D., 1802–1877. (Fig. 2.7)[28], Professor of Midwifery at University College, London, wrote several papers[29, 30] on the use of chloroform in obstetrics and included a chapter in his textbook[31], which was based on his lectures to his students at University College. A

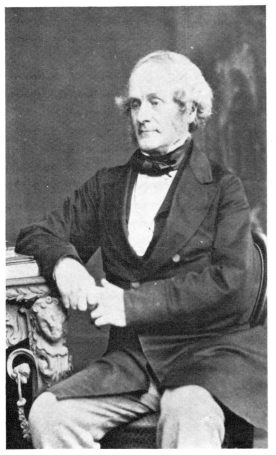

paper of 5 February 1848 was a very early exposition of the use of chloroform in midwifery, and was read to the Harveian Society of London. His pamphlet of 1855 was in effect a defence of the views of James Young Simpson; in it he pointed out that 'man who was destined "to eat bread *in sorrow* all the days of his life", still continued to dine as comfortably as his

means permitted, notwithstanding the curse.' John Snow mentioned that 'Dr Murphy and Dr Rigby were amongst the first to state that relief from pain may be afforded in obstetric cases without removing the consciousness of the patient'[32], thus placing these two obstetricians among those who early recognized the condition of analgesia, though not by that name.

The Murphy inhaler was described in 1848[29]. It consists of a circular metal drum, $1\frac{3}{4}$ in (47mm) in diameter containing a sponge and carrying a circular copper disc inspiratory valve and a silk expiratory flap valve on its upper surface (Figs. 2.8, 2.9, 2.10). To this is soldered a brass mouth-piece (originally cloth or leather covered), the opening between it and the chloroform drum being controlled by a port. 'The nostrils were closed by the fingers until the effect of chloroform was observable, when they were allowed to remain open. The atmospheric air in this way prevented so rapid an action of the vapour as would otherwise take place'[33]. J.R.Pretty of Camden Town stated in 1856, 'the chamber should be charged with about three quarters of a drachm (2.5ml) of chloroform, and it should be held only by the forefinger and thumb, so as not to heat it unduly. The chloroform should be administered so as to diminish or remove suffering—at least almost so—without loss of consciousness and voluntary motion. In this way its use may be continued for several hours with perfect safety. It is made by Mr Coxeter, of Grafton-Street for 6s.6d., or if plated, 12s.6d'[34]. The example in the King Collection, (Fig. 2.8) was made by Stevens and Pratt, Oxford Street, London.

Murphy's inhaler was a neat, compact piece of apparatus, one of the first to appear as an alternative to the use of the 'corner of a towel' advocated by Simpson. Its efficiency cannot have been high, since

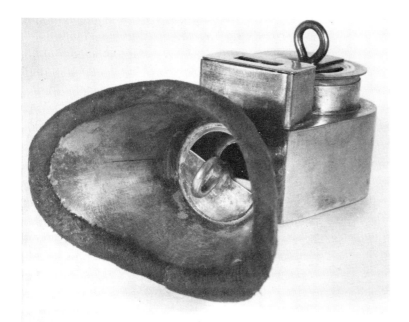

FIG. 2.8. MURPHY'S CHLOROFORM INHALER, 1850.
The openings for inspiratory and expiratory valves are shown. The rim of the face mask is protected with cloth. The main drum holds a sponge and may be closed off by the two rings when not in use. CKC 3

the amount of chloroform allowed was very small and air was admitted freely. Nevertheless it enabled Murphy (and, one hopes, the patient) to appreciate the effect of chloroform analgesia.

FIG. 2.9. MURPHY CHLOROFORM INHALER.
From his book *Lectures on the Principles and Practice of Midwifery.* (1862) p. 576

CKC 11: CHLOROFORM INHALER
c. 1865 (attributed to Sansom)

Arthur Ernest Sansom, M.D., F.R.C.P., 1838–1907[35] (Fig. 2.11) was consulting physician to the London Hospital, and an acknowledged authority on diseases of the heart and lungs. As a student he had seen Snow work at King's College Hospital, and had administered chloroform for William Fergusson[36] and other notable surgeons. He wrote extensively on anaesthesia[36, 37, 38, 39] and his book on *Chloro-*

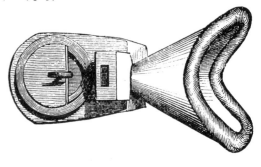

Chloroform inhaler.

CHLOROFORM;

ITS PROPERTIES AND SAFETY

IN

CHILDBIRTH.

BY

EDWARD WILLIAM MURPHY, A.M., M.D.

PROFESSOR OF MIDWIFERY, UNIVERSITY COLLEGE; OBSTETRIC PHYSICIAN,
UNIVERSITY COLLEGE HOSPITAL;
FORMERLY ASSISTANT PHYSICIAN DUBLIN LYING-IN HOSPITAL;
LATE PRESIDENT MEDICAL SOCIETY OF LONDON;
ETC., ETC.

———

" Νήδυμος Ύπνος μὲν κασίγνητος Θανάτοιο."

" Take thou this phial, being then in bed,
And this distilled liquor, drink thou off.
When presently through all thy veins shall come
A cold and drowsy humor, which shall seize
Each vital spirit.   *   *   *
And then awake as from a pleasing sleep."
ROMEO AND JULIET.

———

LONDON:

WALTON AND MABERLY,

UPPER GOWER STREET, AND IVY LANE, PATERNOSTER ROW.
—
M.DCCC.LV.

FIG. 2.10. TITLE PAGE OF MURPHY
on *Chloroform*, 1855.

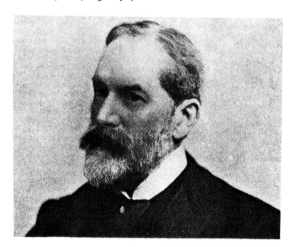

FIG. 2.11. ARTHUR ERNEST
SANSOM, M.D., 1838–1907.

form (1865, Fig. 2.12) also includes records of the use of carbon tetrachloride as an anaesthetic. This book is described by Munk as 'highly practical'[40]. Sansom also wrote The *Antiseptic System*, 1871, supporting Listerism at a time when the work of Pasteur and Lister had not yet received due recognition. In 1861 he described an apparatus for the inhalation of chloroform from a bottle through one nostril, used for excision of the maxilla[38]. The operation was performed by William Fergusson at King's College Hospital, and Sansom stated that the method was a modification of that used by Fauré of Paris[41]. The apparatus consisted of a glass bottle with two tubes, one of which led to a nostril. The other nostril was used as 'a valve to be closed or left open'. The mouth was open and allowed 'sufficient dilution with air.'

Sansom's obituary states 'in all his writings Dr Sansom's earnest desire was to inculcate precision of observation and record.'

Later developments resembling the present apparatus (dated *c.* 1865) are shown by Duncum[41], who describes it as a popular modification of Snow's

chloroform inhaler, and the present model (Figs. 2.13, 2.14) is modified so much from the descriptions that Charles King's original attribution must be held to be tentative, as indeed King realized. Sansom claimed to have improved on Snow's chloroform apparatus (see Duncum, p. 187) chiefly in reducing the chloroform percentage; this he did by making a small metal vaporizing chamber, three inches (8cm) in height, and one and a half inches (4cm) in diameter, and by lining this cylinder with guttapercha which prevented overheating when held in the hand. This notion is greatly in contrast to the principle upheld by Snow, who provided a water jacket for the maintenance of a constant temperature, and thereby, he considered, a constant vapour uptake. Sansom's early models had a perforated cap for the ingress of air, the cylinder was filled with loosely crumpled blotting paper or a roll of lint, and a side tube communicated directly with a face mask or through a wide-bore tube to a nostril tube (Fig. 2.15). The present model has a lint roll vaporizing surface, the delivery tube comes from the upper end, and in place of a perforated cup, a series of numbered air holes is arranged along a metal collar, to correspond to holes punched in the delivery tube. It is thought that the larger hole in the cylinder held an inspiratory valve.

CKC 17/63/A17: JUNKER CHLOROFORM INHALER (1867) AND MODIFICATIONS

Ferdinand Adalbert* Junker was born in Vienna on 7 July 1828. He graduated M.D. at the University of Vienna in 1854 and soon afterwards came to London

* In England, the middle name is given as Edelbert or Ethelbert; his full name was Ferdinand Adalbert Junker von Langegg. Professor Olë Secher of Copenhagen has given valuable help in elucidating the complicated life-story.

CHLOROFORM:

FIG. 2.12. TITLE PAGE OF SANSOM, on *Chloroform*, 1865.

ITS

ACTION AND ADMINISTRATION.

A HANDBOOK.

BY

ARTHUR ERNEST SANSOM, M.B.Lond.,

LATE HOUSE PHYSICIAN, AND PHYSICIAN-ACCOUCHEUR'S ASSISTANT TO KING'S COLLEGE HOSPITAL.

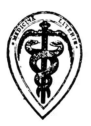

LONDON:

JOHN CHURCHILL AND SONS, NEW BURLINGTON STREET.

MDCCCLXV.

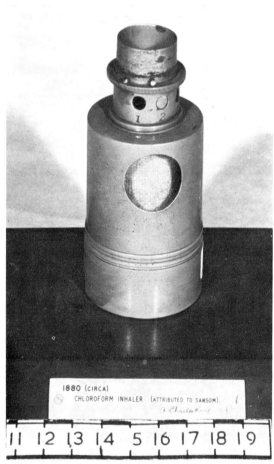

FIG. 2.13. SANSOM CHLOROFORM
INHALER 1880
(attribution by Charles King).
The large opening may have carried
an inspiratory valve. Note the
numbered collar of air entry
perforations. The expiratory valve
was on the face mask.   CKC 11

where in 1860 he became a member of the Royal
College of Surgeons, and was physician to the
Samaritan Free Hospital. In 1870 he returned to
Germany to serve in the Franco-Prussian War, and
became Surgeon-in-Chief of the German Hospital
at Saarbrucken.

In 1873 Junker went to Japan, as chief physician
and Director of the new Hospital and Medical
School at Kyoto. The Japanese had advertised for a
European doctor, preferably German, but English
speaking, who 'must be well versed in the theory and
practice of medicine, and not be a mere theorist or
bookworm. He must learn the Japanese language . . .
a man of good general education, good manners and
kind hearted . . . must love children. He must not
be pedantic, or like a drill sergeant and of temperate
habits. He must be in good health, sound in wind
and limb and eyesight:' their agent in Germany was
also instructed to choose out of two candidates (all
other things being equal) 'the shorter, because, as
they are not a tall people, they would expect more
sympathy from a man who was not tall himself'[42].
This story has been discussed by Thomas[43] and
Matsuki[44].

Since the Japanese had been in contact with the
outside world for only seven years, it is of interest
that they found German medical ways agreeable in
their efforts to modernize their own medicine. Presumably they found the paragon* whom they sought
in Ferdinand Ethelbert Junker, but he remained in
Japan for only four years, and by 1882 was again in
London, where he lived in Hyde Park Gate and presumably practised medicine. He probably died
about 1901, but no obituary notice has been found.

Junker made two significant contributions to
anaesthesia. In 1872, he wrote an important paper

* Matsuki shows that Junker was disliked and mistrusted
by the Japanese.

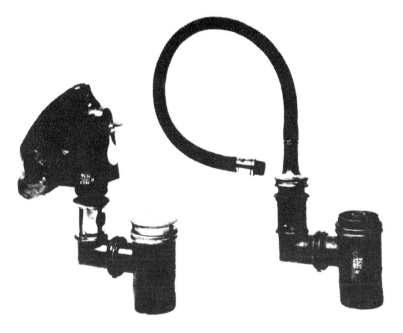

FIG. 2.14. SANSOM CHLOROFORM
INHALER, (*c.* 1865)
as shown in Duncum,B. (1947)
*Development of Inhalation
Anaesthesia* p. 238

on the use of the tracheal tampon, having witnessed the use of a cuffed tracheotomy tube by Trendelenburg in 1872 (see Hahn tube, p. 83). Previously in 1867, he described the Junker bottle, which he used at first with bichloride of methylene, the name given to a physical mixture of chloroform and methyl alcohol. This was first used by Spencer Wells in 1867, and he continued to give it successfully, using a Junker inhaler, for over twenty years.

The Junker inhaler was soon used with pure chloroform and was the most popular apparatus for this purpose, from the time of its introduction to the early years of the present century (Fig. 2.16).

The Junker apparatus was the first to use the 'blow-over' principle, pressure being provided by means of a hand-bellows. Duncum points out that the hand-bellows had been introduced the year pre-

viously by Benjamin Ward Richardson in his ether spray for local analgesia, and it was therefore in the public eye.

In its early design (Fig. 2.17, CKC A.17) Junker's apparatus consisted merely of a graduated bottle which was two-thirds filled with eight drachms (27ml) of liquid. An afferent tube from the bellows led below the fluid and a short efferent tube led the anaesthetic/air mixture through rubber tubing to a vulcanite face piece, which Junker described as having the shape of one half of a hollow spheroid, the rim having notches for the chin and nose, and carrying an expiratory valve on the dome. (see Fig. 2.21).

This model was dangerous. As late as 1927, W.J.Foster was pleading (*Brit. med. J.* 1927. **i**. 261) for the destruction of all valveless models. A fatality

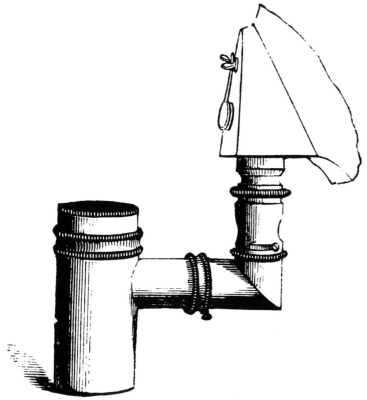

FIG. 2.15. SANSOM CHLOROFORM
INHALER
adapted to the sitting position.
From Sansom, A.E. (1865)
Chloroform. p. 127

had recently occurred at an R.A.M.C. hospital, the apparatus having been incorrectly assembled by a corporal before handing to the anaesthetist! The Coroner's verdict was 'misadventure'. Hewitt had written much earlier of fatalities occurring from coupling the bellows to the efferent tube, and from tilting of the bottle. Modifications were therefore made and two of these may be examined in the collection, in addition to an original Junker bottle (Figs. 2.18 to 2.23). The original manufacturers, Krohne and Sesemann of London, made various improvements and suggested the use of a Skinner's face mask (see CKC 50); they also added a feather indicator to the original expiratory valve; Dudley Buxton of University College Hospital used a foot-pump[45], and sheathed the afferent (inlet) tube within the efferent (outlet) inside the bottle[46]. (Figs. 2.18, 2.19, CKC 63); Kappeler of Munster-lingen invented a modification allowing for the administration of dilute graduated doses, stated to be of known percentages; Frederick Hewitt intro-duced an elaborate but successful innovation by making the afferent tube of large bore and placing the efferent within it. (Figs. 2.20, 2.21, 2.22); a further type has a shortened efferent tube with a ball valve preventing the passage of air should the bellows

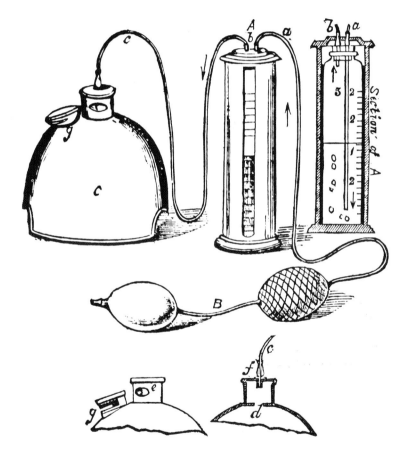

FIG. 2.16. JUNKER CHLOROFORM
INHALER, 1867.
From his original paper
Description of a new Apparatus for
Administering Narcotic Vapours.
Med. Times and Gaz. (1867) **ii**, 590

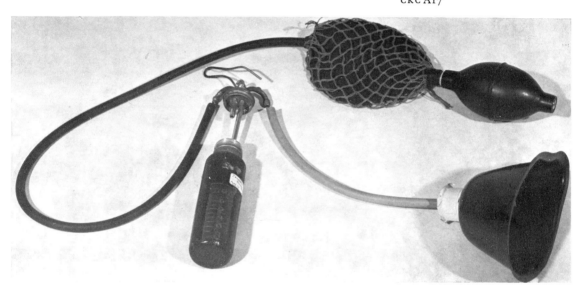

FIG. 2.17. JUNKER BOTTLE IN ITS
EARLY (UNSAFE) STATE.
This provided a new concept in
anaesthesia—the 'blow-over'
principle. The double tube bottle
was however dangerous, as wrong
connection caused the carriage of
liquid chloroform to the patient.
The mask and bellows are modern.
CKC A17

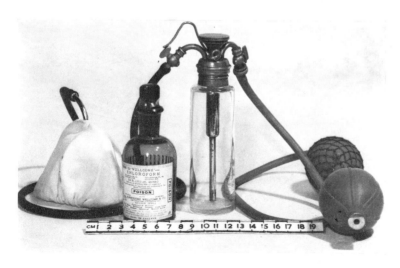

FIG. 2.18. DUDLEY BUXTON'S
MODIFICATION OF JUNKER
INHALER.
The danger of inhaling liquid
chloroform is reduced by enclosing
the longer afferent tube within a
shortened efferent tube, a small gap
between the two acting as the
efferent port. A hook is provided to
hang the bottle vertically from the
lapel. In this specimen the face
mask is original, the bellows being
modern.
CKC 63

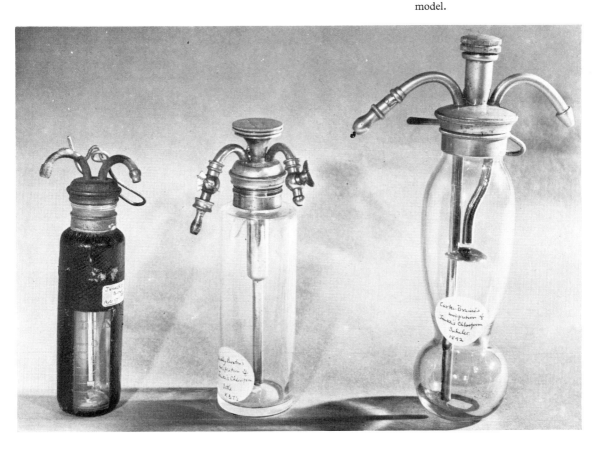

FIG. 2.19. MODIFICATIONS OF
JUNKER BOTTLE.
Left, original 'unsafe' version.
Middle, Dudley Buxton's *c.* 1890.
Right, Carter–Braine's, 1892.
Note the differing tube couplings,
designed to prevent wrong
connection, on the Carter–Braine
model.

FIG. 2.20. HEWITT'S
MODIFICATION OF JUNKER
INHALER. *c.* 1890.
Cf CKC 17. (Fig. 2.17).
The bottle is similar to that of
Dudley Buxton (Fig. 2.18), and has
a clip for vertical support in the
breast pocket—this was satisfactory
till the anaesthetist leaned over!

Incorrect connection of the tubes
was avoided by placing the efferent
tube within the afferent, a somewhat
elaborate modification more
conveniently solved by Carter–
Braine (see Fig. 2.23).
Described in Hewitt,F.
Anaesthetics. 2nd ed. (1901) pp. 316–
318

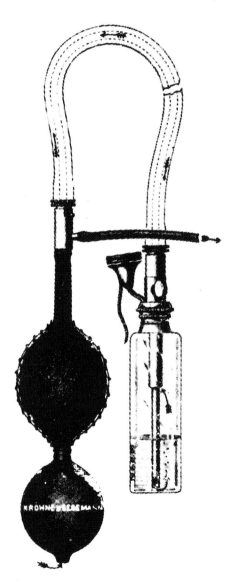

be connected wrongly. All made a point that the
bottle should be hung from the button-hole, and not
removed, even for filling! A hook was provided
(Fig. 2.21). A modification due to Carter Braine is
shown in Figs. 2.19, 2.23.

Masks too were modified, from the original
vulcanite half sphere of Krohne and Sesemann (Fig.
2.21) to a simple lint-on-wire face piece (Fig. 2.18:
CKC 63.) or one of Buxton's which incorporated a
perforated cross-wire in a glass sided cage[47].

Junker's apparatus was mentioned by Geoffrey
Kaye as being in use as late as the Second World
War. Kaye described a version in which a ball valve
was placed on the inlet tube below the surface of the
chloroform, and he wrote in 1942 'Junker's apparatus
and chloroform anaesthesia have fallen largely into
desuetude. Occasion may arise however, and
especially in field units, when the apparatus may be
turned to good account. Its use will be so familiar to
the reader that a detailed description is scarcely
required'[48].

A further use for Junker's apparatus was found by
Sir Francis Shipway, who placed a bottle in his
warmed ether/chloroform system from 1916 onwards
(see CKC 25, 26, p. 182).

There is no doubt of the value of Junker's inhaler
to the anaesthetists of the 1870's and 1880's, particularly for work inside the mouth, when a tube or gag
was connected to the bottle (Figs. 2.24, 2.25); but it
had its limitations, and Frederick Hewitt stated
these—'It is practically impossible to say what
percentage of chloroform vapour is usually inhaled . . . (it) will depend on a variety of circumstances. Foremost of these is the quantity of air
taken up with each inspiration. . . . The next most
important factor is probably the manner in which
the face piece fits or the degree to which air gaining
admission through it when it is adapted accurately

to the features. Then we must take into account the temperature of the chloroform at the time: and this will greatly depend upon the rapidity with which the air is forced through the liquid. Professor Zengerle of Constanze conducted, at Kappeler's request, some interesting experiments on this point. I reproduce his figures[49].

Experiment	Compression of Bellows per minute.	Quantity of Air supplied.	Chloroform evaporated.
I	120	4 litres	.7 gm
2	60	2.2 litres	1.2 gm
3	40	1.6 litres	1.4 gm
4	30	1.2 litres	1.5 gm
5	24	1.0 litres	1.6 gm
6	20	.9 litres	1.7 gm
7	17	.8 litres	1.7 gm
8	15	.7 litres	1.7 gm

Temperature of chloroform 63.5°F (17°C)

From these experiments it is concluded that the speed of pumping is in inverse ratio to the percentage of chloroform in the issuing air. The temperature of the room will also exert a slight influence. But, although the percentage of chloroform vapour must vary widely . . . the following calculation may give an idea of the percentage inhaled. Given that the respiration of the patient is unimpeded: that he breathes at the rate of 24 per minute: that he inhales 540cu in (9 litres) of air per minute (Lister): that the bellows of the inhaler are compressed only during each inspiration, so that all the chloroform vapour is inspired: and that 1 grain (60mg) of chloroform produces .767cu in (12.5cc) of vapour at 60°F (16°C) (Snow): then applying Zengerle's table an atmosphere of 3.5% of chloroform vapour will be

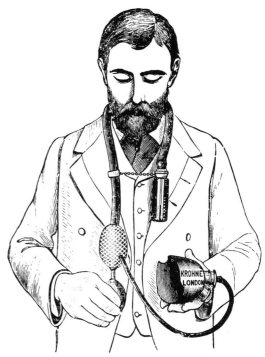

FIG. 2.21. HEWITT'S MODIFICATION OF JUNKER INHALER.
As worn by the smart anaesthetist.

breathed by the patient. In this calculation it is taken for granted that all the chloroform evaporated by each pump of the bellows is inhaled. Should the face piece fit loosely, some would escape, and the same would occur if the pumping were not accurately timed with inspiration, when the percentage would be less than 3.5. On the other hand should the breathing be shallow, and not more than 200cu in (3.2 l) of air be inspired per minute, a considerably higher, and possibly a dangerous, percentage of vapour would result'[50].

This passage written by Hewitt in 1901, affords an interesting glimpse of the state of experimental anaesthesia at that time.

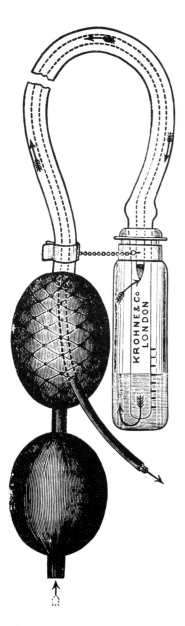

FIG. 2.22. FURTHER
MODIFICATION BY HEWITT OF
JUNKER INHALER.
This model has a shortened efferent
tube.
Described in Hewitt,F.
Anaesthesia. (1893) p. 195

CKC 6: HAHN TUBE AND TAMPON,
with Trendelenburg cone, for chloroform after
tracheotomy 1871

Wilhelm Friedrich Hahn 1796–1874, practised in
Stuttgart. Friedrich Trendelenburg, 1844–1924 (Fig.
2.26), of Berlin, is best known for his surgical work,
for example, his operation for ligature of the
saphenous vein for varicose veins, (1890) and the
first pulmonary embolectomy in 1908. This was unsuccessful, but he lived just long enough to see a
successful embolectomy performed by his pupil
Kirschner in 1924. The Trendelenburg position for
operating on the viscera was described in 1881.

Hahn's tracheotomy tube (Fig. 2.27, CKC 6) consisted of a curved metal tube, 6cm in length and
8mm in diameter, covered with sponge. A flanged
plate allowed the tube to be tied in place and its
orifice was connected to an angle piece which in turn
connected to a narrow bore tube originally 60cm or
more in length, at the distal end of which was
attached a conical funnel—Trendelenburg's cone
(Fig. 2.27). Chloroform was dropped on to a piece
of domette stretched across its open end. The
original cone had a ring of holes below the cover,
through which air was drawn. (Figs. 2.28, 2.29).
Trendelenburg also modified the tracheotomy tube
by substituting an inflatable rubber cuff for the
sponge (Fig. 2.30). This tampon cannula was
introduced in 1869 for the treatment of tracheal
stricture by tracheotomy.

In 1909 Probyn-Williams wrote 'In some extensive
operations in the mouth . . . tracheostomy is first

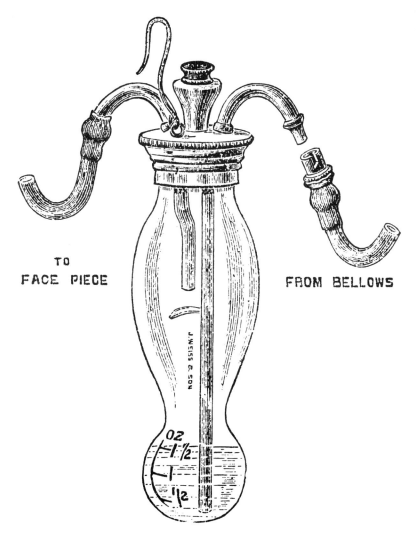

TO
FACE PIECE

FROM BELLOWS

FIG. 2.23. CARTER BRAINE'S
MODIFICATION OF JUNKER
INHALER.
The upper bulb of the bottle has
three times the capacity of the
lower, and the egress tube is fixed
in the centre of the larger bulb.
Chloroform cannot therefore be
driven over. Splashing is prevented
by a flange attached to the longer
tube. Changing the tubes is
impossible as one has a bayonet
catch, the other being plain.
See Carter Braine. (1892) A Safety
Junker Inhaler. *Brit. med. J.* **i**, 1364.

FIG. 2.24. BENT METAL MOUTH-
TUBE
for use with Junker Inhaler.
From Hewitt, F. *Anaesthetics*.
(1893) p. 199

FIG. 2.25. MASON GAG WITH
CHLOROFORM TUBE ATTACHED
for use with Junker Inhaler.
From Hewitt, F. *Anaesthetics*.
(1893) p. 200.

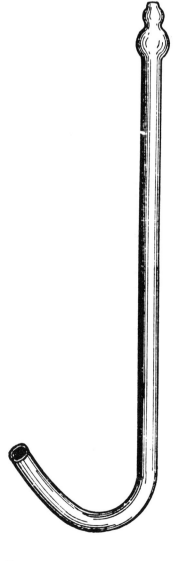

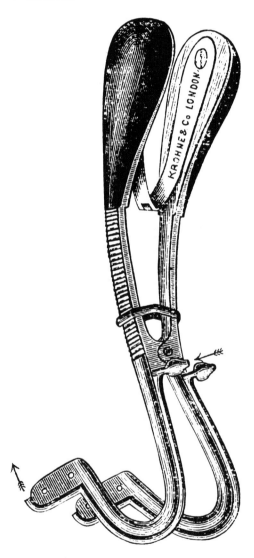

performed, and then chloroform is administered through the tracheostomy tube. Blood is prevented from entering the trachea by packing the pharynx with sponges or by means of a small bladder round the tracheostomy tube which is inflated (Trendelenburg's tampon) or by a sponge round the tube which absorbs the blood till it swells and so blocks the trachea (Hahn's tube)'[51]. (Fig. 2.31.)

Boyle, 1907, recommended the use of Hahn's tube for thyrotomy and excision of the larynx. This was advanced surgery for its period, but the problems met with, particularly when using a plain laryngotomy tube, were stated by Boyle—'any bubbling noise in the tube or the onset of cyanosis will probably indicate that there is excessive mucus in the trachea or that blood has trickled past the sponge. Such events are met by . . . passing a feather down the tube to remove the blood or mucus. It is sometimes a good plan to suspend the administration for a few minutes in order that the depth of anaesthesia may be so far diminished as to allow the trachea to be cleared by coughing. The anaesthetist must then be ready with a sponge to remove the blood and mucus coughed up, otherwise it will be drawn in again by the next inspiration'[52]. In these circumstances, it seems strange that anaesthetists were so long in demanding suction apparatus as a standard part of their equipment.

Hewitt[53] commented on the same problem and preferred to use a Skinner's mask (see CKC 50) instead of the Trendelenburg cone, as blood and mucus were more easily removed, or coughed out, from the open end of the tracheotomy tube. He used the Trendelenburg tube only when the respiration was quiet and the colour good. Later Hewitt preferred to use a Junker apparatus to pump chloroform vapour down a small silk catheter passed down the tracheotomy tube. He also used the Trendelen-

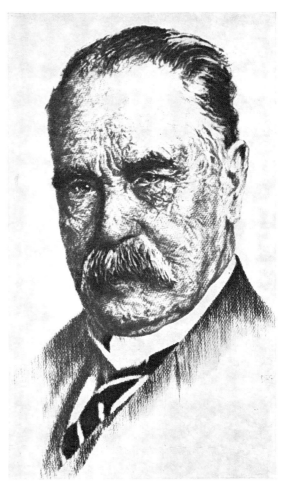

FIG. 2.26. FRIEDRICH TRENDELENBURG, 1844–1924, Berlin surgeon best known for his operating position and for his advocacy of pulmonary embolectomy.

FIG. 2.27. HAHN
TRACHEOTOMY TUBE WITH
TRENDELENBURG
CHLOROFORM CONE.
The sponge cover for the
tracheotomy tube is shown. The
original connecting tube was longer
(60cm) than in this specimen, and
was wire-wound. The
Trendelenburg cone was originally
described with a row of air holes.
These appear to have been omitted
in later models. (See Fig. 2.28)
CKC6

FIG. 2.28. TRENDELENBURG
CONE, AS FIRST DESCRIBED IN
1869.
The row of air holes is shown. Their
later omission might have been a
retrograde step, but perhaps was
dictated by a need for respiration to
take place through the chloroform-
impregnated domette. The
Trendelenburg tampon was inflated
with air by a separate balloon, and a
pilot was provided. (See Fig. 2.30.)

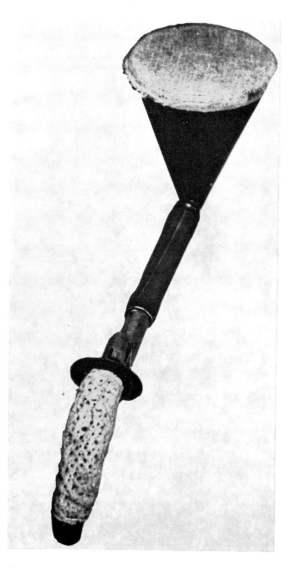

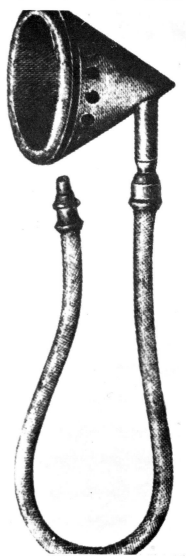

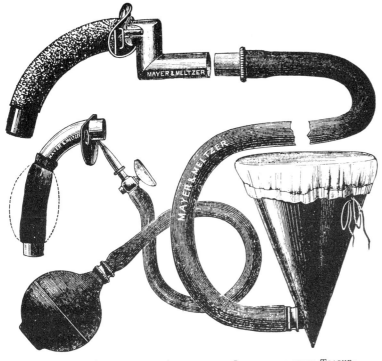

FIG. 2.29. BOTH HAHN AND
TRENDELENBURG TUBES ARE
SHOWN,
together with the inflating bulb and
chloroform cone.
From Probyn-Williams,R.J. (1909)
*Practical Guide for the
Administration of Anaesthetics.*
p. 156

APPARATUS FOR ADMINISTERING CHLOROFORM AFTER TRACHE-
OTOMY. The upper tube with sponge is known as Hahn's, the lower, with a
bag which is inflated with air, is Trendelenburg's.

burg head down position[54].

Hewitt found that the Trendelenburg balloon gave better results than Hahn's sponge, saying that he knew of one or two cases in which the latter allowed the passage of blood into the trachea.

The important work was that of Trendelenburg, who in 1869 had concluded that packing of the trachea was a vital part of all operations on the larynx and pharynx. He thus evolved the technique of tracheotomy, following chloroform induction, with the subsequent introduction of his cannula with

a tampon—'a delicate double-walled india rubber tube of about 3–4 centimetres in length' which was then inflated 'through a small tube opening into the external wall' by means of 'a small india rubber balloon with an ivory nozzle'[55] (Figs. 2.29, 2.30). F.E.Junker (see page 71) reported on two cases, one with a maxillary tumour 'of gigantic proportions' which he had seen operated upon by Professor Langenbeck in Berlin, in 1872[56]. Trendelenburg used his tracheotomy tube after preliminary anaesthesia with chloroform. Langenbeck com-

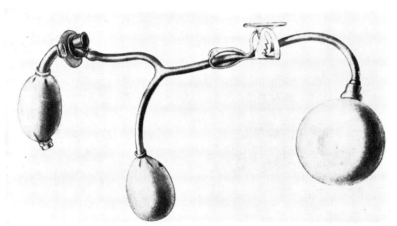

FIG. 2.30. TRENDELENBURG
TAMPON CANNULA AND
TRACHEOTOMY TUBE,
with inflating and pilot balloons,
developed from the tube first
described in 1869.
From Kirschner. (1931) *Operative
Surgery*.

mented that 'he would not in future perform any operation on the face, in which inspiration or deglutition of blood may be apprehended, without using Dr Trendelenburg's instrument'. This opinion of a great surgeon is justified in Junker's paper, which discusses the physiology and application of the technique in a very interesting essay.

The Hahn tube, particularly as it was adapted by Trendelenburg, was an important advance on the slow road to endotracheal anaesthesia.

CKC 20: VERNON HARCOURT CHLOROFORM INHALER 1903

Augustus George Vernon Harcourt[57], F.R.S., 1834–1919 (Fig. 2.32) was Reader in Chemistry, Christ Church College, Oxford. He was a pioneer in what was then the new science of physical chemistry and greatly endeared himself as a teacher to generations of students. Between 1899 and 1911 he was concerned with the administration of chloroform. In 1899 he devised a means for estimating the percen-

FIG. 2.31. HAHN SPONGE
TRACHEOTOMY TUBE.
The tightly bound tape was
removed immediately before use.
The moisture of the trachea then
caused it to swell.
From Kirschner, (1931) *Operative
Surgery*. p. 156.

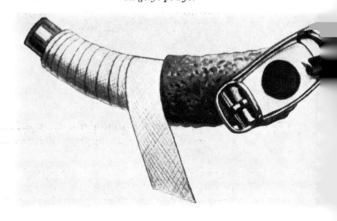

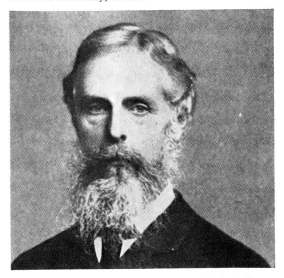

tage of chloroform in air, by converting the chloroform into carbon dioxide and hydrochloric acid in
contact with a red-hot platinum wire in the presence
of steam, and of water to absorb the hydrochloric
acid.

Vernon Harcourt's work was so intimately connected with investigations into the physiology and
practice of chloroform anaesthesia, and with the
Chloroform Committee of 1901, that it is necessary
here to discuss the background to the setting up of
that Committee and its work. In Montreal in 1897,
Dr A.D.Waller, F.R.S., (see p. 92) Lecturer in
Physiology at St Mary's Hospital, London, and
later Director of the Physiology Laboratory of the
University of London, read a paper to the Annual
General Meeting of the British Medical Association
in which he maintained that the deaths due to
chloroform were avoidable and unjustifiable[58]. In
1898 he returned to the subject when speaking to the
Society of Anaesthetists, saying that 'successful
chloroform anaesthesia requires the regular respiration of air in which the chloroform vapour is maintained between the limits of 1 and 2 per cent'[59]. In
1901 Waller wrote a letter to the Council of the
British Medical Association (published with the
Committee's Report in 1910 [60] in which he said
that 'deaths are in the overwhelming majority of
cases due to overdosage.' He suggested the setting
up of a committee of investigation into the action of
chloroform.

Such a committee was set up in 1901, a distinguished panel of experts forming the body, of whom
the medical members included Waller himself, as
first Chairman, Professor Charles Sherrington,
F.R.S., Sir Victor Horsley, F.R.S., and the anaesthetists Dr McCardie, of Birmingham, and Dr
Dudley Buxton, of University College Hospital, who
acted as secretary. Vernon Harcourt was a co-opted
member.

The objects stated were to 'investigate methods of
quantitatively determining the presence of chloroform in the air and in the living body' and, on a
more practical level, 'to determine if possible, what
is the minimal dose of the drug which would secure
adequate anaesthesia for operations and at the same
time not endanger life'[60]. The Committee sat for 9
years and produced a long and comprehensive report
in 1910 running to some twenty-five pages of the
journal. The physiology of respiration and absorbtion of chloroform was described and earlier attempts
at precise chloroform dosage e.g. Duroy's anaesthesiometer, 1856, and the experiments of Paul Bert
in the 1880's were mentioned. The main object of
the committee was to find a safe dosage and the

FIG. 2.33. VERNON HARCOURT
CHLOROFORM INHALER, 1903.
The mixture control is set at 0.5 per
cent. Beneath the chloroform bottle
is a warming candle. The face mask
has an expiratory valve.
The apparatus was made by
Messrs. Griffin & Co., of Kingsway,
London.
CKC 20

means of attaining it.

Goodman Levy[61], B.J.Collingwood[62], and others designed regulatory inhalers which were described and investigated; among these others were Dr Waller himself (CKC 61) and Vernon Harcourt, whose inhaler appeared in 1903. His colleagues described this as having 'the advantages of simplicity, exactness and portability' and they adopted it in their experiments. The inhaler (Fig. 2.33) is said to provide an automatic mixture with a maximum strength of two per cent, and this can be diluted at will with air[63]; some anaesthetists did not believe in the exactness of the percentage obtained, and criticized the length of time taken for induction[64].

The following extracts from the report describe the design. The double-necked glass bottle (Fig. 2.34) is filled with chloroform and two glass beads act as temperature indicators. If the temperature of the liquid chloroform is below 16°C. both beads will float; if it is above 18°C. both will sink;* in the former case the proportion of chloroform inhaled will be less than indicated; in the latter case, it will be higher. Cooling by evaporation is countered by warming the bottle until the beads begin to sink (the specimen shown carries a candle on a stand!) The dimensions of the bottle are carefully designed, the diameter of the upper portion having been proportioned to the average rate of human respiration and to the rate of evaporation of chloroform between 16°C. and 18°C. To compensate for varying rates of respiration the inlet and outlet of the bottle are placed near together and at some distance from the surface of the liquid, while to compensate for the lowering of the liquid surface by evaporation the vessel widens to its base. The nearness of the two

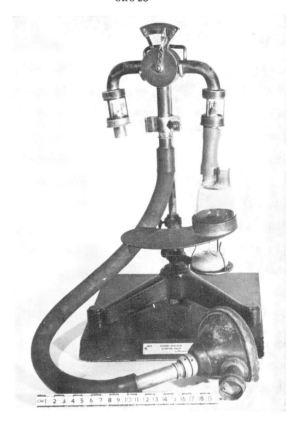

necks and the distance from them to the surface of the chloroform, diminish the variation in the proportion of inhaled air to that of chloroform vapour which is caused by shallow or deep breathing, the latter producing a lowered chloroform percentage and vice versa. It is stated that 'if the rate of breathing is voluntarily reduced to 3 l a minute instead of 7 l, the proportion of chloroform may be raised to about 2.5 per cent.' If respiration is raised above 7 l, the proportion falls to 1.5 per cent. The stopcock

---

* In some bottles, the red bead floated while the blue sank, at the specified temperatures.

FIG. 2.34. THE GLASS
CHLOROFORM BOTTLE
showing the two wide-bore, closely
set necks, and the tapered form
which compensates for lowering of
the liquid surface as the chloroform
evaporates.
From Buxton,D. (1914)
Anaesthetics. p. 244

FIG. 2.35. MIXTURE CONTROL OF
THE VERNON HARCOURT
CHLOROFORM INHALER,
set at 0.5 per cent. When set to
2 per cent air is admitted only via
the chloroform vaporizing bottle.
(Cf. Fig. 2.33, in which the scale
is read from right to left).

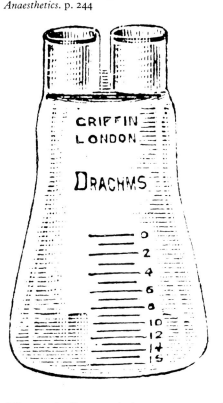

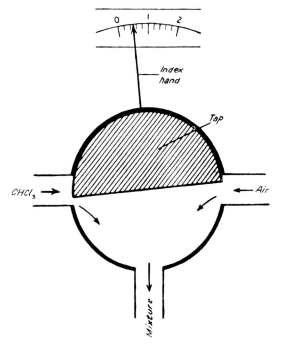

(Fig. 2.35) allows variations up to a maximum of 2 per cent and it is claimed that for maintenance of anaesthesia a dose of one per cent or less is sufficient. It is apparent that allowance must be made for fall of temperature or agitation of the liquid.

The metal unidirectional valves (Fig. 2.36) are very light and are arranged so that 'only one valve opens when the pointer is at either end of the scale, both equally when the pointer is midway, and for other positions proportionately, depending upon the position of the pointer'.

The apparatus could be used suspended from the anaesthetist's neck (Fig. 2.37), or mounted on a stand (Fig. 2.38). Pages 69–72 of the Report of 1910[60] are occupied by a detailed description of the Vernon Harcourt inhaler in use written by Dr Dudley Buxton, secretary of the Committee, who also described it in the fifth edition of his textbook on anaesthetics[65]. More than one member of the Committee, it is said, actually took chloroform using Vernon Harcourt's apparatus. Buxton described its use in children, in adults, the aged, and in unusual difficulties, and the consensus was decidedly in favour of this type of inhaler.

'The Committee' reads the report 'determined to accept the two per cent vapour of chloroform as a

FIG. 2.36. VERNON HARCOURT
METAL UNI-DIRECTIONAL VALVE
mounted in a glass expansion of the
tubing.

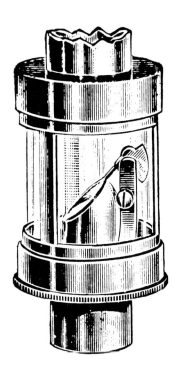

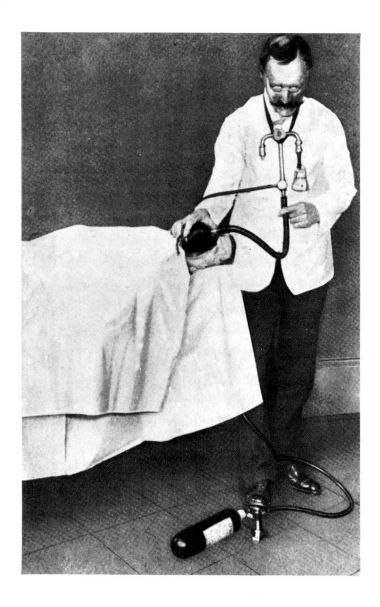

FIG. 2.37. VERNON HARCOURT
CHLOROFORM INHALER IN USE.
In this instance, a foot-controlled
oxygen cylinder is connected,
oxygen being delivered through a
side-tube on the patient's side of the
mixing control.
From Buxton, D.W. (1914)
Anaesthetics. pl. v.

sufficient maximal dose for adults during the induction period, and therefore suggested that limit as the maximum on the scale of the Vernon Harcourt inhaler. To exceed this . . . is dangerous. The safest method is that which leaves least to chance, and this is believed to be found in a dosimetric inhaler with a maximal delivery of a two per cent vapour'. But 'the machine must remain a machine and demands that the user shall possess knowledge and adequate skill'.

The popularity of the Vernon Harcourt Inhaler is indicated by its description (usually taken directly from the Report) in all the major textbooks of the period: Gwathmey of New York commented favourably and included a photograph of the apparatus[66]. Some however, such as Blomfield and Carter Braine, complained of the length of time taken in induction. McCardie took an average of sixteen minutes over induction using a one per cent setting. The inhaler seems to have had a short life and probably failed to survive the Great War partly owing to its delicacy and partly to the fall in popularity of chloroform as the deaths continued.

Unfortunately the lack of understanding of the true physiology of the action of chloroform persisted. Embley from the Physiological Laboratory of the University of Melbourne in 1902, insisted that vagal inhibition in dogs was the 'great factor in the course of sudden death under chloroform'[67].

In 1911, Goodman Levy gave the answer. Commenting that restriction of chloroform dosage by percentage had failed to reduce the incidence of death, Levy in a classic series of demonstrations, showed that ventricular fibrillation occurred in chloroformed cats and that an exactly similar form of death could be reproduced by injecting small doses of adrenalin into a cat lightly anaesthetized with chloroform[68] (See Fig. 2.6).

Goodman Levy dealt the final blow to chloroform, though anaesthetists were slow to recognize this. There are no references to adrenalin in the presence of chloroform in Bellamy-Gardner, 1916[69], in Gwathmey[70] or other works of the period. However, Hadfield[71] mentions Levy and his work in 1935, and the 1923 edition of Boyle and Hewer[72] states that primary cardiac failure can occur with chloroform 'when adrenalin is injected or applied to a cut surface'. There is no mention of Levy, light anaesthesia or endogenous adrenalin. Gwathmey (p. 373) even states, though without reference, 'Delbet has adminstered adrenalin to more than 1,000 chloroformed patients. The results have been splendid. He believes that adrenalin regularises the narcosis and diminishes post-operative shock'.

The Committee on Anaesthesia of the American Medical Association of 1912, stated that 'the use of chloroform for major operations is unjustifiable,' but chloroform had been little used in America. A qualified view is expressed by Stuart Ross, 1919, 'so far as the author understands the views of Dr Levy, his explanation of chloroform syncope need not be taken as introducing any new principle into the administration of the drug'[73]. However, Ross does warn against the use of adrenalin in surgery. Waters and Meek[74] showed the effect of chloroform in reducing the refractory period, with increasing liability to ventricular fibrillation. Gradually the facts became a canon of anaesthetic lore and chloroform slowly passed from use.

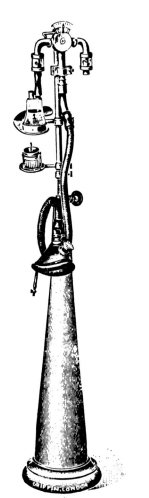

The Vernon
Harcourt chloroform re-
gulator. The index in-
dicates 1 per cent.

The inhaler is shown fixed
to a stand with an arrangement for warming the
chloroform

CKC 61: WALLER CHLOROFORM BALANCE. 1903. MODERN REVISION BY E.J. & J.W.C.FOX 1968.

Augustus Desiré Waller, M.D., F.R.S., 1856–1922[75] (Fig. 2.39) was lecturer in Physiology at St Mary's Hospital, London; later he became Director of the Physiological Laboratory of the University of London and Dean of the Faculty of Science. An exact and inventive experimental physiologist, he has important claims to attention from the anaesthetist, for he was the first to demonstrate the action currents of the heart, and in 1887 obtained the first electrocardiogram in man[76, 77], using the mirror galvanometer and the capillary electrometer. This long predated the discoveries of Einthoven who perfected the string galvanometer in 1901. The development of electrocardiography was due to Waller's pioneering, though it was a consequential finding resulting from a general investigation of the electric potentials in living structures, especially in nerves and muscles, and in the skin and retina. For this work he was elected F.R.S. at the early age of thirty-six.

Waller was brought up in an environment of physiology. His father, Augustus Volney Waller, 1816–1870, was professor at Birmingham, whose demonstration of the law of nerve degeneration in 1850 gave his name to this phenomenon, the starting point of the 'neurone theory'.

The younger Waller was born in Paris, receiving his early education there. He became interested in the use of chloroform as a laboratory tool and in anaesthesia when making observations on the effects

FIG. 2.39. AUGUSTUS DESIRÉ WALLER, F.R.S., 1856–1922; obtained the first electrocardiogram in 1887. He insisted that the danger of chloroform depended on the percentage of vapour in the inhaled air.

A gay and eccentric personality, his home was used as a laboratory to the extent that the exigencies of space required the billiard table to double also as a working bench and a dining table!

The bulldog was used by Waller in his experiments. Jimmie stood 'in a state of voluntary immobility' with legs in glass vessels containing saline while electrocardiographs were made. Questioned in the House of Commons about cruelty, Mr Gladstone answered 'I have made the acquaintance . . . of the dog, who is well accustomed to these exhibitions and likes standing in the water' (*The Times*, 9 July 1909).

When Waller married a biscuit heiress, Miss Palmer of Reading, his students wrote on his blackboard 'Waller takes the biscuit'. His riposte was 'and the tin as well', and his wife's fortune enabled him to continue in physiological research for the remainder of his life; but he always regarded physiology as the servant of clinical medicine.

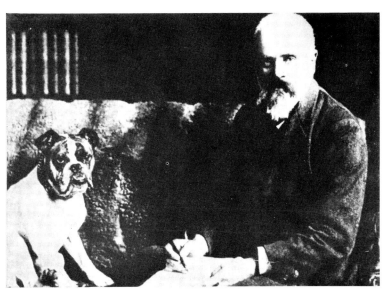

of gases and anaesthetics on the irritability of nerve-muscle preparations (Fig. 2.40). Observing that the effect of ether on the electrical state of a nerve is reversible, whereas that of chloroform is to kill, Waller wrote[78]—'This experiment has caused me much thought. It seemed to me to represent, as in a nutshell, anaesthesia of the human subject. It was a rough-and-ready experiment representing in the laboratory, the sort of thing that can happen in rough-and-ready practice, when the vapour of ether or of chloroform is used—carefully, perhaps—but with very indefinite knowledge of their strength or of the quantity absorbed. I then thought it very probable that chloroform accidents ascribed to "idiosyncrasy" might in reality be due to overdose'. Here Waller referred to no less than thirteen papers written by himself between 1897 and 1909 on topics related to chloroform anaesthesia. He went on 'I

thought that we required above all, more precise knowledge of power and quantity. Yet today, although I hear less about idiosyncrasy and more about actual quantity and percentage, I still recognise an excessive disposition to invoke any cause other than simple overdosage to account for fatal accidents', including '*status lymphaticus*'. He continued 'obviously the first question to be studied in the laboratory, for its own sake and for the sake of the hospital, is the question of quantity, a question of most pressing importance as regards chloroform. How much chloroform is required to produce anaesthesia? How much chloroform is dangerous or assuredly fatal? How shall we best administer the smallest sufficient quantity of chloroform?

'These are eminently practical questions that require to be answered by careful experiments in the physiological laboratory, completed by careful

FIG. 2.40. WALLER'S DIAGRAM OF
THE EFFECTS OF ETHER AND
CHLOROFORM
upon the electrical state of nerve.
There is no recovery from
chloroform. The percentages of the
drugs used are not stated; it was
early days for such investigations.
From Waller,A.D. (1910)
Physiology, the Servant of Medicine.
p. 32

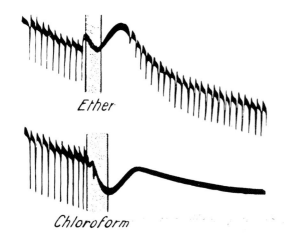

Ether

Chloroform

observations in the hospital. And so I was led to make experiments on the isolated tissues of animals, and on animals themselves—on isolated nerve, on the spinal cord, on isolated muscle, on the heart, on blood-pressure—that have little by little brought out what to my mind are clear and satisfactory answers, both as regards the smallest sufficient quantity required, and as regards simple methods of determining such quantity, as well as of regulating it during administration. I wanted to indicate how the laboratory and the hospital have business together in ways that might not have been anticipated. I for one did not do so when I first etherised a nerve to see whether its response was physiological or not'.

These and similar quotations are engrossing material for the anaesthetist and Waller's little book is worthy of careful perusal.

As a result of the knowledge which he had thus acquired, and, as he says, of the need for laboratory and hospital to 'have business together', Waller, in 1901 initiated the Special Chloroform Committee of the British Medical Association which was set up under his chairmanship in the same year and finally reported in 1910[79]. The findings of this Committee and its effects upon the use of chloroform, have already been discussed (see p. 85). As has been shown, many percentage inhalers were investigated, including those of Waller himself, for he devised two forms, the *wick inhaler* and the *Balance Inhaler*, which is represented by a model now at Abingdon (Figs. 2.41, 2.42). It is described thus: (Fig. 2.43) 'air is pumped by a small electric motor through an ordinary wide-mouthed bottle containing liquid $CHCl_3$ into a large mixing chamber of 30 l capacity, containing the balance and provided with an inlet from the bottle and an outlet to the tube and face-piece. The flow of air is rendered uniform and of suitable volume per minute by means of an elastic reservoir and a perforated stop on the course of the supply tube. The percentage of the mixture is watched on the pointer attached to the beam of the balance. When the case contains air only the counter-poise is slightly the lighter of the two, and the index points to 0. When the mixture of air and chloroform passes into the balance case, the bulb being far larger than the solid metal counterpoise and therefore displacing more of the gas around, it loses more of its weight when the density of the mixed gases increases and therefore the index moves over the arc to a position determined by the density of the mixed gases.'

'The percentage is regulated by varying the depth of a tube in the chloroform bottle and by admitting more air. The chamber can be placed at any distance from the patient. As the inhaler is made on the plenum system, no respiratory difficulty arises through the length of the supply tube. An addition can be made by which a permanent record can be made of the strength of the vapour given throughout

FIG. 2.41. WALLER CHLOROFORM
BALANCE, 1903.
Specimen housed at Penlon Ltd.,
Abingdon. Property of the Nuffield
Department of Anaesthetics,
Radcliffe Infirmary, Oxford.

This balance was perhaps used for
animal work. The bulb is of
500cu cm and the case capacity is
20 litres. The counter-poise weighs
20gm. Controls on left for
admission of chloroform vapour,

with outlet to patient on lower
right. Displacement of the bulb in
chloroform vapour allowed direct
measurement of the percentage by
movement of the balance arm.

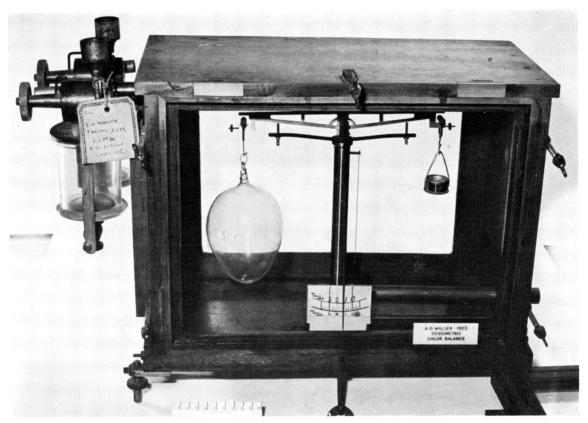

the narcosis. The inhaler has been employed in some cases for surgical anaesthesia and with success. In its present form however, it is hardly applicable for everyday surgical use. The accuracy of its delivery has been tested and the nominal percentage can be maintained with some degree of accuracy'[80]

Waller's balance was originally described for use on the laboratory animal. In his book *Physiology, the Servant of Medicine,* the glass bulb is shown as having a capacity of 250cu cm as also in Waller's

original diagram (Fig. 2.43). The Report of the Special Committee shows a bulb of 870cu cm while Dr Fox gives 1,000cu cm[81]. The capacity of the chamber is given in both earlier instances as 30 l. In the only original model available these measurements are approximately 500cu cm and 20 l (Fig. 2.41).

In 1968, Drs John and Elizabeth Fox of the State University of New York, demonstrated at the Fourth World Congress of Anaesthesiologists, in London, their modern revision of the Waller chloroform

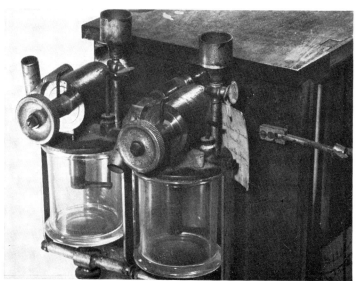

balance (Fig. 2.44). The mixing chamber of perspex
contains a 'bulb' made by glueing together two
plastic cups (capacity 300ml) and the beam activates
an electronic balance from which a direct chloroform
percentage may be read on a scale. This model was
presented to the Charles King Collection by the
Doctors Fox, whose paper is included in the proceedings of the Congress, under the title *The Waller
Chloroform Balance Revisited*[81]. Dr John Fox who
read the paper, described his apparatus as consisting
of a piezo-transistor, in which weight from a 'globe'
formed of two plastic cups, was applied to the top
of the transistor to modify its shape. Suitable
electronic pick-up enables the voltage energy change
to be metered. Fox commented that the signal-to-
noise ratio greatly modified the weight-signal
generated, particularly by the lower concentrations
and he speculated that Waller too might have been

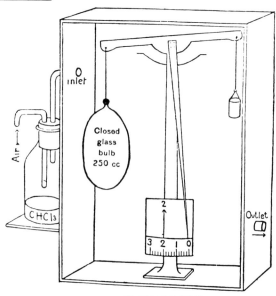

The Chloroform Balance.

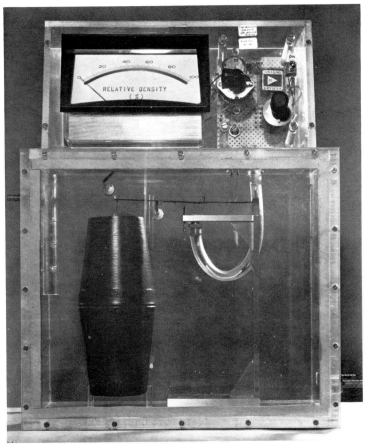

FIG. 2.44. WALLER CHLOROFORM
BALANCE REVISITED.
Electronic version made by
Dr J.W.C.Fox and Dr Elizabeth
Fox, New York.
Presented to the Charles King
Collection, 1968.
The beam carries a 'globe' made
from two plastic cups, and is
connected via a piezo-transistor to
the recorder.
CKC 61

harassed by excessive swinging of the balance at each input of vapour. In fact, Waller comments that a light recording pen fixed to the beam of the balance, and a smoked cylinder, apart from making a record, served also to damp the oscillations of the beam and pointer. He also used a large volume vessel (30 l) for the mixture, as this avoided accidental fluctuations in the percentage of chloroform delivered. It is evident that in the Fox revision as it stands, the electronic form is too sensitive to induced changes. Waller's original model might have been of greater practical application, though its bulk and lack of portability were disadvantageous.

FIG. 2.45. HIRSCH CHLOROFORM
INHALER.
Diagram from paper to *Lancet*.
1916. **i**. 730
A—Air-inlet, closed.
B—Chloroform wick round central
tube.
C—Wick around wall of chamber.
F—Chloroform tube.
G—Baffle plate.
H—Chloroform by-pass to air tube.

CKC 27: HIRSCH PERCENTAGE CHLOROFORM INHALER 1916

Charles Theodore William Hirsch, L.S.A., M.R.C.S., L.R.C.P., 1869–1927 was educated at the London Hospital and became anaesthetist to the Samaritan Hospital, London, which had also been Junker's hospital, and to eight other hospitals in London. He was a keen and early motorist and for many years, he wrote weekly articles for the *Lancet* on motoring matters[82]. He evidently turned this activity to good account, for this apparatus was manufactured for him by Mr Cliff, motor engineer, of Well Hall, Kent.

In 1916, Hirsch described this inhaler[83] (Figs. 2.45, 2.46) and claimed an accurate percentage reading, verified by Professor Waller on his chloroform balance. His description of the apparatus shows it to have provided a simple draw-over through the central air tube, 15mm in diameter, into which the chloroform vapour is drawn through a by-pass (H) (Fig. 2.45) Hirsch wrote 'as the port is opened, chloroform vapour is drawn through the by-pass in the same way as air is sucked into a Bunsen burner'[84]. The drum capacity is about 85cu ml and the measured amount of chloroform, 12 drachms (= 40cu ml) is placed therein. No bag was used and Hirsch claimed complete absence of rebreathing.

The rotating collar is graduated from zero to 3.5 per cent. 'In use it is found advisable to start with the port closed, indicator at zero, and to take five to ten minutes in passing gradually to 2.5%, when surgical anaesthesia is generally produced. A higher percentage is rarely needed'. 'The expirations of the patient maintain a constant temperature in the chloroform chamber, and from actual experiments at that temperature the dial on the lid is graduated to show the percentage being inhaled'[83].

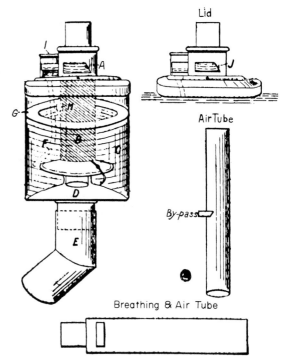

These statements seem optimistic, and though he recognized the work of Levy, and viewed chloroform with caution, Hirsch was able to write 'Chloroform is said to be the most dangerous of all anaesthetics—I question this. The personal factor applies, and with care and attention I believe it is safe: other anaesthetists think otherwise. Some go so far as to say it is criminal to use it'[83].

These remarks were addressed to an audience of students and others at the National Dental Hospital, University College Hospital, London, and were printed in 1925, fourteen years after the work of Goodman Levy! Hirsch claimed 10,000 chloroform

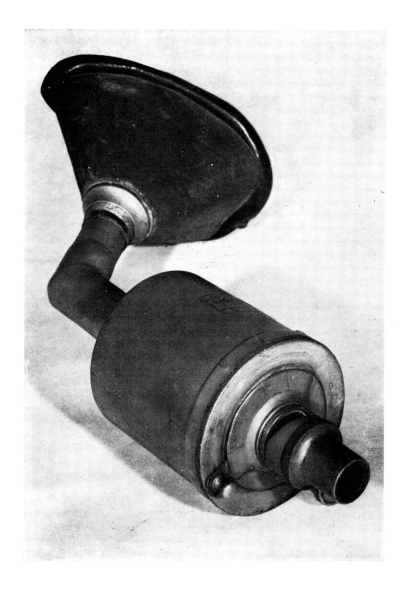

FIG. 2.46. HIRSCH PERCENTAGE
CHLOROFORM INHALER, 1916.
The variable air-intake may be seen
with the revolving collar graduated
from zero to 3.5 per cent.
CKC 27

The expiratory valve is seen to the
side of the mask, which lacks its
rubber rim. The upper container
holds the chloroform sponge.
CKC 70

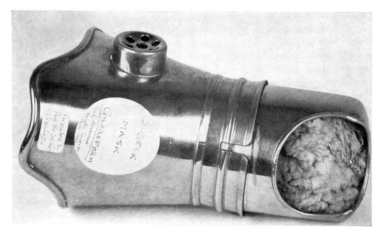

anaesthetics without a death but had had three
deaths under ether[84], of which he gave no further
details. Hirsch's apparatus is an early attempt to
make use of the Venturi principle.

CKC 70: SUDECK CHLOROFORM INHALER, c. 1900

Paul Herman Martin Sudeck 1866–1938, Professor
of Surgery in Hamburg, produced this inhaler, to
which a tentative date of 1900 is here given. The
specimen was kindly donated by Professor Olë
Secher, Copenhagen, who also provided some
biographical detail. Three eponyms are associated
with Sudeck; i. his critical point, the junctional
avascular region on the colon between the supplies
of the colic and superior rectal arteries; ii. Sudeck's
osteoporosis and iii. Sudeck's paresis[85].

The chloroform inhaler consists of a metal face
piece (originally with a rubber rim) shaped to fit
over nose and mouth. (Fig. 2.47). It tapers distally
to a wide collar of 2 in (5cm) diameter which is

closed by a fixed metal diaphragm in the centre of
which a mica inspiratory valve is placed. On the side
of the face piece is a similar expiratory valve. (Fig.
2.48). Into the collar may be fitted a cylindrical
metal sponge container some $2\frac{1}{2}$ in (6.5cm) in
height, which has a large eccentric hole in its upper
part, into which the sponge is passed.

In use, the two parts were assembled, chloroform
was poured on to the sponge, and the mask firmly
fitted to the face; inspiration took place through the
impregnated sponge and through the connecting one
way valve, the expired vapours passing out through
the side valve on the face-piece. No details are
known as to the amounts of chloroform used, and in
practice, the apparatus would have provided a portable, though uncontrolled, method of administering
chloroform, with a probably unacceptable degree of
oxygen limitation and carbon dioxide accumulation.
No references to its construction or use have been
found.

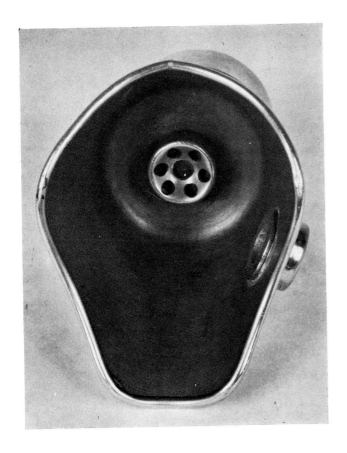

FIG. 2.48. SUDECK INHALER,
interior of face piece to show
inspiratory and expiratory valves.

REFERENCES

1 SIMPSON J.Y. (1847) *Account of a new anaesthetic agent as a substitute for sulphuric ether in Surgery and Midwifery.* Edinburgh: Sutherland and Knox.

2 SIMPSON EVE (1896) *Sir James Y. Simpson.* Edinburgh: Oliphant, Anderson and Ferrier. p. 58.

3 THOMAS K.B. (1971) The Early Use of Chloroform. *Anaesthesia.* **26.** 348.

4 SIMPSON J.Y. (1848) *Answer to to the Religious Objections advanced against the Employment of Anaesthetic Agents in Midwifery and Surgery.* Edinburgh: Sutherland and Knox.

5 TOMES J. (1848) *Dental Physiology and Surgery.* London: Parker. p. 349.

6 COOK H. (1847) Surgical Operations performed by the inhalation of chloroform. *Lancet.* **ii.** 571.

7 DUMAS M.J. (1834) Chloroforme. *Annales de Chimie et de Physique.* **56.** 115–120.

8 SNOW J. (1858) *On Chloroform and other Anaesthetics.* London: Churchill. p. 112.

9 SNOW J. (1858) *ibid.* p. 217.

10 SNOW J. (1858) *ibid.* p. 251.

11 SNOW J. (1858) *ibid.* p. 261.

12 SNOW J. (1858) *ibid.* p. 260.

13 DUNCUM B. (1947) *Development of Inhalation Anaesthesia.* London: Oxford Univ. Press. p. 226.

14 SNOW J. (1858) *op. cit.* p. 251.

15 JUNKER F.E. (1872) On the Use of the Tracheal Tampon. *Med. Times & Gaz.* **i.** 510.

16 Obituary notices: (1915) Edward Lawrie, M.D. *Lancet.* **ii.** 581. *Brit. Med. J.* **ii.** 350.

17 MASSON A.H.B., WILSON J., HOVELL B.C. (1969) Edward Lawrie of the Hyderabad Chloroform Commission. *Brit. J. Anaesth.* **41.** 1002.

18 THOMAS K.B. (1974) Chloroform Commissions and Omissions. *Proc. Roy. Soc. Med.* **67.** 723–730.

19 LISTER J. (1909) *The Collected Papers of Joseph, Baron Lister.* Oxford: Clarendon Press. p. 149.

20 WOOD H.C., HARE H.A. (1890) The Cause of Death from Chloroform. *Medical News.* (Feb. 22). Philadelphia.

21 GASKELL W.H., SHORE L.E. (1893). Report of the Physiological Action of Chloroform: with a criticism of the Second Hyderabad Commission. *Brit. Med. J.* **i.** 105. 164. 222.

22 McWILLIAM J.A. (1890) Experimental Investigation on the Action of Chloroform and Ether. *Brit. Med. J.* **ii.** 831. 890. 948.

23 LEVY A.G. (1922) *Chloroform Anaesthesia.* London: Bale and Danielsson.

24 COLLINGWOOD B.J. (1905) An Apparatus for the delivery of Chloroform Vapour of known dilution. *Med. Chir. Trans.* **88.** 695.

25 LEVY A.G. (1911) Sudden death under light chloroform. *J. Physiol.* **42.** iii.

26 ROOD F.S. & WEBBER H.N. (1930) *Anaesthesia and Anaesthetics.* London: Cassell, p. 129.

27 Editorial (1972). *Brit. J. Anaesth.* **44.** 909.

28 Obituary notices: (1877) E.W. Murphy. *Lancet.* **i.** 111. *Brit. Med. J.* **i.** 99.

29 MURPHY E.W. (1848) *Chloroform in the practice of midwifery.* London: Harveian Society.

30 MURPHY E.W. (1855) *Chloroform, its Properties and Safety in Childbirth.* London: Walton and Maberley.

31 MURPHY E.W. (1852). *Lectures on the principles and practice of Midwifery.* London: Walton and Maberley. (2nd ed. 1862).

32 SNOW J. (1858) *On Chloroform and other Anaesthetics.* London. p. 318.

33 MURPHY E.W. (1848) *op. cit.* p. 14.

34 PRETTY J.R. (1856) *Aids during Labour.* London: Churchill, p. 72.

35 Obituary notice: (1907) A.E. Sansom. *Lancet.* **i.** 843.

36 SANSOM A.E. (1865). *Chloroform its actions and administration.* London: Churchill. preface.

37 SANSOM A.E. (1869) *Anaesthetics in obstetric practice.* London: Churchill.

38 SANSOM A.E. (1861) Administration of chloroform by the nostril in operations on the mouth. *Med. Times and Gazette.* **i.** 550.

39 SANSOM A.E. (1865) *op. cit.* pp. 148. 184.

40 *Munk's Lives of the Fellows of the Royal College of Physicians of London* (1955). London: Royal College of Physicians., vol. IV. p. 260.

41 DUNCUM B. (1947) *op. cit.* p. 238.

42 *Med. T. & Gaz.* 1872. i. 740.

43 THOMAS K.B. (1973) Ferdinand Edelbert Junker. *Anaesthesia.* **28.** 531–534.

44 MATSUKI F. (1974) Junker in Japan. *Anaesthesia.* **29.** 607–609.

45 BUXTON D.W. (1888) *Anaesthetics, their Uses and Administration.* London: Lewis. p. 76.

46 BUXTON D.W. (1900) *Anaesthetics.* 3rd ed. London: Lewis. p. 176.

47 DUNCUM B. (1947) *op. cit.* p. 472.

48 KAYE G. (1942) *Manual of Army Anaesthetic Apparatus.* Australian Military Forces. Melbourne. p. 50.

49 KAPPELER O. (1880) *Anaesthetica: Deutsche Chirurgie* **20.** 142.

50 HEWITT F.W. (1901) *Anaesthetics and their Administration.* London: Macmillan. 2nd ed. p. 318.

51 PROBYN-WILLIAMS R.J. (1909) *A Practical Guide to the Administration of Anaesthetics.* London: Longmans, Green. 2nd ed. p. 155.

52 BOYLE H.E.G. (1907) *Practical Anaesthetics.* London: Hodder and Stoughton. p. 158.

53 HEWITT F.W. (1893) *Anaesthetics and their Administration.* London: Griffin. p. 41.

54 HEWITT F.W. (1901) *op. cit.* p. 148.

55 DUNCUM B. (1947) *op. cit.* p. 599.

56 JUNKER F.E. (1872) On the use of the Tracheal Tampon. *Med. Times & Gaz.* i. 510. 595.

57 Obituary notice (1920) A. Vernon Harcourt. *Proc. Roy. Soc.* Series A. **97.** *vii.*

58 WALLER A.D. (1897) Action of Anaesthetics upon Nerve: Ether and Chloroform. *Brit. med. J.* ii. 1469.

59 WALLER A.D. (1898) The Dosage of Anaesthetics. *Trans. Soc. Anaesth.* i. 78.

60 Report of Special Chloroform Committee (1910) *Brit. Med. J.* **ii.** Supp. pp. 47–72.

61 LEVY G. (1904) (On Chloroform) *Lancet.* ii. 1496.

62 COLLINGWOOD B.J. (1910) An Apparatus for the delivery of chloroform vapour of known dilution. *Brit. med. J.* **ii.** Supp. 67.

63 VERNON HARCOURT A.G. (1903). Special Chloroform Committee *Brit. Med. J.* **ii.** Supp. p. 142.

64 HAMMES T. (1904) The Harcourt Inhaler. *Brit. Med. J.* **ii.** 1118.

65 BUXTON D. (1914) *Anaesthetics, their uses and Administration.* London: Lewis. pp. 243–251.

66 GWATHMEY J.T. (1905) The Vapour Method of Anesthesia. *Medical Record.* **68.** 609.

67 EMBLEY E.H. (1902) The Causation of Death during the the Administration of Chloroform. *Brit. Med. J.* **i.** 817. 885. 951. 975.

68 LEVY, A. GOODMAN (1911) *op. cit.*

69 GARDNER H. BELLAMY (1916) *Manual of Surgical Anaesthesia.* Toronto: Macmillan. 2nd. ed.

70 GWATHMEY J.T. (1914) *Anaesthesia.* New York: Appleton.

71 HADFIELD C.F. (1935) *Practical Anesthetics.* London: Ballière, Tindall & Cox.

72 BOYLE H.E.G. & HEWER C.L. (1923) *Practical Anaesthetics.* London: Hodder & Stoughton. 3rd ed. p. 105.

73 ROSS J.S. (1919) *Handbook of Anaesthetics.* Edinburgh: Livingstone. p. 113.

74 WATERS R.M. et al. (1951) *Chloroform. A Study after 100 Years.* Univ. of Wisconsin Press. p. 53 et seq.

75 Obituary notice: (1922) A.D. Waller. *Brit. Med. J.* **i.** 458.

76 WALLER A.D. (1887) A demonstration in man of electromotive changes accompanying the heart's beat. *J. Physiol.* London. **8.** 229.

77 WALLER A.D. (1910) *Physiology, the Servant of Medicine. Chloroform in the Laboratory and in the Hospital: The Hitchcock Lectures for 1909, delivered at the University of California.* London: Univ. of London Press. p. 12.

78 WALLER A.D. (1910) *ibid*.
p. 32–35.

79 Report of Special Chloroform
Committee (1910) *Brit. Med. J.*
ii. supp. pp. 47–72.

80 Report (1910) *ibid*. p. 67.

81 Fox J.W.C. & Fox E.J. (1970)
*Progress in Anaesthesiology.
Proceedings of the Fourth World
Congress of Anaesthesiologists.*
(1968) Amsterdam. Excerpta
Anaesthesiologica. p. 225.

82 Obituary notice: (1927) C.T.W.
Hirsch. *Lancet*. **ii**. 301.

83 HIRSCH C.T.W. (1916) A
Simple Percentage Chloroform
Inhaler. *Lancet*. **i**. 730.

84 HIRSCH C.T.W. (1925) *A Chat
on Anaesthetics*. London: John
Bale and Danielsson, p. 36.

85 DOBSON J. (1962) *Anatomical
Eponyms*. Edinburgh:
Livingston. p. 198.

Section III
The Nitrous Oxide Series

ILLUSTRATIONS

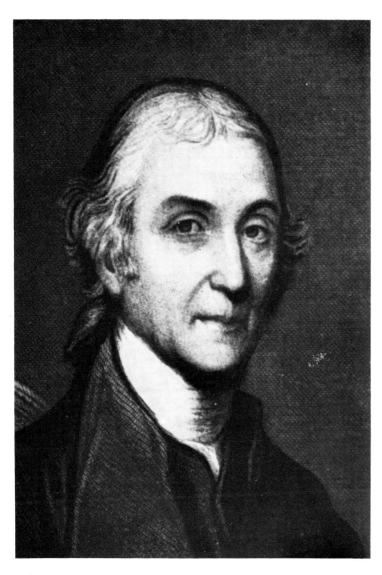

FIG. 3.1. JOSEPH PRIESTLEY,
1733–1804,
who first produced nitrous oxide in
1772.

INTRODUCTION: *THE DISCOVERERS*

The use of nitrous oxide as an anaesthetic came about as the result of many factors. The discovery and the description of the gas by Priestley (Fig. 3.1) in 1772 and 1774 have been ably described by Denis Smith[1]. Gaseous and vapour therapies were well-beloved activities of physicians and patients in the latter part of the eighteenth century and it is hardly to be wondered at that this extraordinary new gas, which was respirable, which supported combustion but which did not support life, should take its place alongside oxygen, which had also been isolated by Priestley and Scheele in the 1770's, as a panacea for many ills. As Priestley himself wrote of oxygen 'who can tell that, in time, this pure air may become a fashionable article in luxury. Hitherto only two mice and myself have had the privilege of breathing it'[2]. Priestley's prediction proved true. Doctors, fashionable and obscure, orthodox and quack, soon became fascinated by these new 'airs'.

The Pneumatic Institution

Among the more interesting of these physicians was Thomas Beddoes, 1760–1808 (Fig. 3.2) who obtained his medical doctorate from Oxford and then forsook medicine for chemistry, becoming Reader from 1788–92. He was a man of original ideas and out-spoken nature, and students flocked to his lectures, but his radical and liberal notions were too vigorous for the conservative Oxford common room; in 1793, after expressing candid and sympathetic views on the French Revolution, Beddoes left for Clifton, where he worked for some years as a leading exponent of pneumatic medicine; here in 1799, he opened the Pneumatic Medical Institution, (Fig. 3.3)

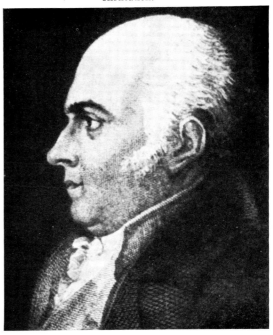

FIG. 3.2. THOMAS BEDDOES, M.D., 1760–1808
founder of the Bristol Pneumatic Institution.

designed for the study of the use of gases in medicine, where patients would be treated freely with these new substances.

Beddoes was a prolific and varied writer. His views on pneumatic medicine are proclaimed in the Brunonian statement—'that diseases of excitement on the one hand, and debility on the other might be cured by a proper air one can hardly doubt'[3]. That he had made a study both of the discovery and introduction of gases, and of the function of respiration, is shown by his translation of the works of the seventeenth century physiologist John Mayow, who

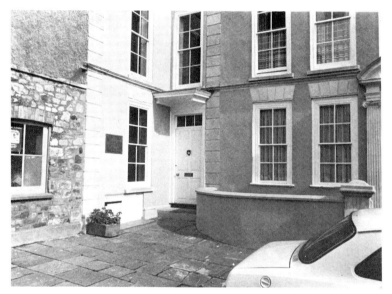

FIG. 3.3. THE BRISTOL
PNEUMATIC INSTITUTION IN 1974.
No. 6, Dowry Square, Clifton, used
by Humphry Davy as his laboratory.
A plaque erected by the Bristol
Civic Society, records Davy's
researches on nitrous oxide. No. 7,
a portion of whose entrance is
shown, was used for the reception
of patients. (See also Cartwright,
F.F., (1951). p. 102[7]

had foreshadowed the discovery and properties of oxygen[4], and by his reading of a remarkable book by Edmund Goodwyn, M.D., Edinburgh, 1759–1829, entitled *The Connection of Life with Respiration*[5]. Goodwyn showed for the first time that oxygen was removed from the inhaled air, and that carbon dioxide was added. The oxygen thus added to the blood was thought to 'give it a stimulating quality by which it is fitted to excite the left auricle and ventricle to contraction.' Obstruction of the respiration as by drowning thus prevented this exchange of oxygen and the loss of its stimulating effect upon the heart caused the latter to die. Beddoes stated that the writings of Mayow and Goodwyn 'led me to reflect with peculiar earnestness upon the action of the atmospheric air upon the blood'[6]. Beddoes was, however, credulous and impulsive. Cartwright, who gives an excellent account of his life and his Institution,[7] regards him as one who invariably argued from the particular to the general. This, coupled with a poetic mind, a taste for lampoonery and a certain showmanship, caused him to publish, for example, *A New Method of treating Venereal disease by nitrous acid*, (actually nitric acid). In this curious commentary the dedication is made *To Broken Gamblers, Attorneys off the Roll and Footmen out of Character*[8].

Humphry Davy, the young Superintendent (Fig. 3.4)

Beddoes contribution to the story of anaesthesia lies in his appointment of the young Humphry Davy as Superintendent of the Pneumatic Institution, and his employment of James Watt, the greatest engineer of the century, to manufacture the apparatus. Watt had a consumptive son, Gregory, who had been

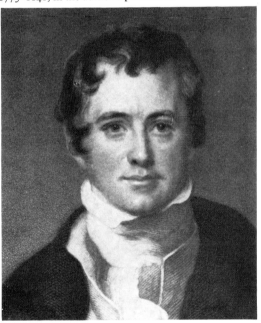

under treatment by Beddoes, and James Watt, impressed by the physician's knowledge of pneumatic medicine, was willing to come to his aid in designing apparatus which was made at the Birmingham factory of Boulton and Watt. It may truly be said that Watt, with his associates, such as William Clayfield, was the original designer of much of our modern anaesthetic apparatus, from retorts, furnaces and 'refrigatory' for the manufacture of gases, to the containing gasometer, the tubing and

the oiled silk bags from which inhalation took place. These were all described in the book which Beddoes and Watt jointly produced in five parts between 1794 and 1796[9] (Fig. 3.5).

Humphry Davy came to the Pneumatic Institution as superintendent in March 1799, at the age of 20; he was described by Beddoes as 'equal to my wishes and superior to my hopes'[10]. Davy had been apprenticed to John Bingham Borlase, surgeon of Penzance. He does not appear to have been the ideal apprentice, but he commenced a course of self-instruction in chemistry in the winter of 1797–98, using primitive apparatus, and reading Nicholson's *Dictionary of Chemistry* and Lavoisier's *Elements of Chemistry* as his guides. The latter greatly excited his interest, but his chief experiments while at Penzance were analyses of air contained in bladder-wrack, and upon light and heat, on which he published an extraordinary theory, a work which he later bitterly regretted. The chance for removal from this life of rural innocence came when he met Davies Giddy (Gilbert), 1767–1839, an amateur but keen and knowledgeable scientist, later to be President of the Royal Society as Davy's successor in that office. Giddy allowed Davy the use of his library at Tredrea near Penzance and it was here that the lad first made the acquaintance of the works of the other chemists, including Priestley and Beddoes. Here too he discovered a paper on nitrous oxide. Davy's own comment was 'a short time after I began the study of chemistry, in March 1798, my attention was directed to the dephlogisticated nitrous gas of Priestley, by Dr Mitchill's theory of Contagion'[11]. Samuel Letham Mitchill was Professor of Chemistry in the College of New York; he put forward the curious theory that nitrous oxide was the principle of contagion, a gas formed by decomposition, and the cause of fever and plague. Davy seized upon this

FIG. 3.5. WILLIAM CLAYFIELD'S
APPARATUS
for the production and storage of
nitrous oxide, *c.* 1798. *A* is the
retort in which the gas was
generated by heating ammonium

nitrate. This and the associated
experimental machinery, were
manufactured by the great
engineering firm of Boulton and
Watt.

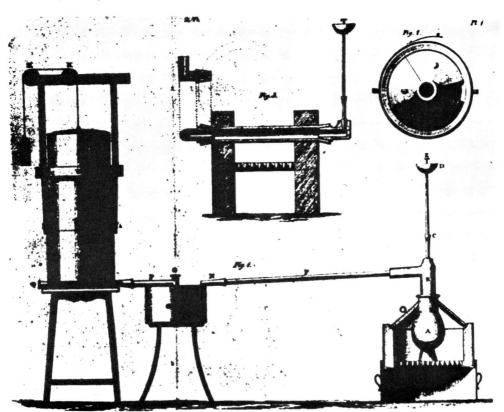

notion, burning with the idea of proving or disproving it. He manufactured very impure nitrous oxide by the action of nitrous acid on zinc. Animals with and without wounds were placed in the gas and Davy himself inhaled it. He wrote to Beddoes, who already had some knowledge of the young apprentice through Gregory Watt; for by coincidence, young Gregory had lodged with Davy's mother while wintering in Cornwall. Later, when Beddoes was seeking his superintendent, the recommendation of

Davies Giddy proved sufficient for Davy to obtain the post which was to lead him to the Royal Institution and eventually to the Presidency of the Royal Society. At Bristol his work consisted in a complete investigation of nitrous oxide, and in 1800 he published the great book *Researches* which brought him much fame, the work of a mere youth, a youth whose whole career in research had been covered in less than two years, the work of a genius. But life was not all work at Bristol. Beddoes was himself no mean poet and Davy's poetic gift was such that Coleridge is said to have remarked that if he had not been the first chemist, he would have been the first poet, of the age. Samuel Taylor Coleridge and Robert Southey were his confidants, Mrs Beddoes was a source of 'gaiety and good humour', and her father Richard Lovell Edgeworth, occasionally added a note of eccentricity, humour and ingenuity. Among other inventions was his plan for a 'telegraph' from Newmarket, so keen was he to know the result of a race!

Many of these, and others, assisted in Davy's experiments, and inhaled nitrous oxide. Southey made a niche for himself in the history of anaesthesia by his note to Davy that he supposed 'the atmosphere of the highest of all possible heavens to be composed of this gas.' This remark, quoted by Beddoes, was picked up forty years later by Gardner Quincy Colton in Connecticut, and provides a distinct link between the work of Davy and the introduction of nitrous oxide into anaesthesia. The recent reproduction edition of Davy's *Researches* has enabled anaesthetists at last readily to read this astonishing book in which the properties of nitrous oxide, chemical, physical and physiological, were minutely investigated, and the well-known remarks were made regarding the effect of the gas on Davy's painful wisdom tooth and on the diminution of physical pain during surgical operations[12].

Davy did not follow up these ideas. His mind was running on other lines, and in 1801 he was appointed as lecturer in chemistry and director of the laboratory to the Royal Institution, London. The Pneumatic Institute lingered on for a few years, but the death of Thomas Beddoes in 1808 put an end to this curious and interesting medical experiment.

It is however, difficult to understand why Davy's idea did not take root. His book was well received and widely read, and his experimental work was commented on and copied in such institutions as the Chemical Class at Guy's Hospital. Yet no one was there to accept the idea of painless surgery and mankind was to suffer for another forty years. As Denis Smith remarks, 'the stage was set but the actors went away.' But perhaps it was not so surprising, if we consider Davy's experiments. In August, 1798, Davy very nearly killed himself by inhaling 'hydrocarbonate', manufactured by the decomposition of water by charcoal. This would produce what we should now call 'water-gas'-carbon monoxide and water. Davy's comment was 'I have been minute in the account of this experiment, because it proves that hydrocarbonate acts as a sedative. . . . There is every reason to believe that if I had taken four or five inspirations instead of three, they would have destroyed life immediately'[13]. Who would have had the temerity to repeat this or any other of Davy's experiments, after such comments ?

Forty Years On

During the next forty years numerous references were made, both to the gas and to ether. In America, and to a smaller extent in England, students very soon made use of the drugs in their *frolics*. In 1808, William Barton of Philadelphia took the nature of the gas as a subject for his doctoral thesis[14]. Ten years later, the journal of the Royal Institution carried a short article in which it was stated—'when the vapour of ether mixed with common air is inhaled, it produces effects very similar to those occasioned by nitrous oxide.' The soporific effect was mentioned, for 'it is necessary to use caution in making experiments of this kind. By the imprudent inspiration of ether, a gentleman was thrown into a very lethargic state, which continued with inter-

FIG. 3.6. HORACE WELLS, 1815–
1848,
first to make use of nitrous oxide for
pain relief. His public demonstration
at Boston in January 1845 was a
failure.

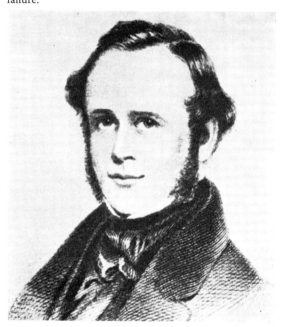

missions for more than thirty hours. . . .'[15] This
note has been attributed to Michael Faraday, but
there seems to be no direct evidence that he was its
author.

The gas was also used therapeutically by many
physicians. This period has been well reviewed by
W.D.A.Smith who writes—'these glimpses of
nitrous oxide are enough to let us see that, in the
United Kingdom it was introduced into the medical
student's curriculum in at least some of the hospitals,
very early in the century: that its preparation was

demonstrated and that it was sometimes inhaled at
lectures on chemistry. It was also inhaled for both
private and public entertainment and doctors knew
sufficient about nitrous oxide to consider using it
therapeutically'[16].

Anaesthesia attained

Nitrous oxide came finally into anaesthesia through
its use by itinerant showmen, and the story of its
introduction to Horace Wells (Fig. 3.6) by Gardner
Quincy Colton (Fig. 3.7) is too well known to need
further telling[17]. In discussing the White nitrous
oxide bag (see Fig. 3.12), we shall discover a possible
cause of the failure of poor Wells in his public
demonstration at the Massachusetts General Hospital
in 1845. Following this failure, nitrous oxide
disappeared from the anaesthetic scene for some
eighteen years.

Its use was continued for the purposes of public
hilarity by Colton during this period, but by 1867
he claimed over 24,000 successful dental administrations at his New York Dental Institute, which he
had founded in 1862. General interest was not
aroused until he demonstrated nitrous oxide
anaesthesia at the International Exhibition in Paris
in 1867. At once the enthusiasm of an influential
American dental surgeon was stirred. Thomas
Wiltberger Evans, 1823–1897 (Fig. 3.8), had worked
in Paris for many years, and his fashionable clientele
included the august person of the Emperor Napoleon
III himself. Among the later adventures of Thomas
Evans, we hear of his part in assisting the Empress
Eugénie to escape from Paris to London in 1870. But
Evans was no dilettante. Within a few months he had
used nitrous oxide in over 1,000 cases, and had
decided that his English colleagues should receive
its benefits, presumably because it was not appreci-

FIG. 3.7. GARDNER QUINCY COLTON, 1814–1898, travelling showman, and founder of the New York Dental Institute, whose continued faith in nitrous oxide was responsible for its reintroduction as an anaesthetic nearly twenty years after Horace Wells' failure. Colton never omitted to give Wells due credit for his original observation that the gas prevents pain.

FIG. 3.8. THOMAS WILTBERGER EVANS, 1823–1897, American dental surgeon working in Paris, whose enthusiasm established the use of nitrous oxide in England in 1868.

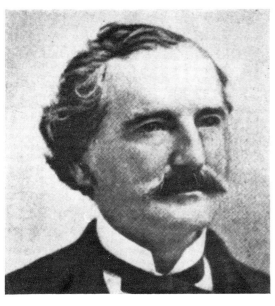

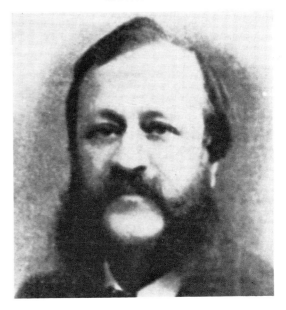

ated by the French! In March 1868, he travelled to England, set up his Sprague generator in his room at the Langham Hotel, filled his gas-bags and gave a demonstration at the surgery of a leading London dentist, David Hepburn, followed by a series at the National Dental and other hospitals.

Though there had been a brief revival of interest in England in 1862, when Samuel Lee Rymer had used the gas (see p. 117), the death of a 'fine young woman'[18], and the difficulties of administration with the apparatus then available, caused both dentists and doctors to turn away once more from its investigation and improvement.

In 1868, however, the English dentists, Alfred Coleman, (see Fig. 2.5) C.J.Fox and others took up the new technique, and though Clover at first expressed his doubts he soon realized that his own chloroform bag provided a ready means of administering gas. (see Fig. 1.10).

The inventive genius of Clover was soon responsible for improvements in apparatus. The supplemental bag and stopcock appeared, Clover stressing the importance of preventing the entry of air (see p. 115).

The introduction of the pressure cylinder was of major importance. In early days, the gas was piped direct from the retort and reservoir (Fig. 3.9). Then came low pressure storage cylinders and finally Messrs. Coxeter in August 1868 produced an apparatus through which the gas might be inhaled direct from the cylinder. Duncum gave an excellent picture of these activities and remarked 'this apparatus was important in that it was the basic model for similar apparatuses during the rest of the

FIG. 3.9. PIPED NITROUS OXIDE,
c. 1890.
In the later nineteenth century,
nitrous oxide was piped into the
dental surgery from the reservoir in
a workshop. The retort and
purifiers are also shown.

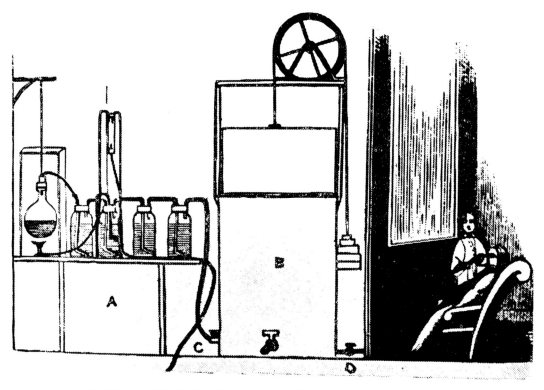

nineteenth century.' (Fig. 3.10)[19]. For further information on this period the papers of Denis Smith should also be consulted[20, 21].

In 1876, Clover introduced his ingenious nitrous oxide/ether apparatus, the first sequential form (see CKC 7, p. 121).

Gas and Oxygen

Though Paul Bert in Paris in the 1860's had conducted experimental and practical work upon the use of nitrous oxide under pressure, and upon the value of oxygen, and though Edmund Andrews of Chicago had shown in 1868 that nitrous oxide anaesthesia was improved by the addition of oxygen, neither of these pioneers received contemporary support, though other workers used methods of compression and a few tried adding oxygen[21].

It was not however, till oxygen became available, like nitrous oxide, under compression in metal cylinders, that progress was possible. The pioneers in this work were the manufacturers, Messrs Coxeter of London and S.S.White of Philadelphia. There is some evidence that S.S.White had bottled oxygen

FIG. 3.10. THE DEVELOPED MODEL
OF THE COXETER NITROUS OXIDE
APPARATUS, *c.* 1890
showing Cattlin reservoir bag, with
a Clover supplemental bag, and his
stopcock and face piece.

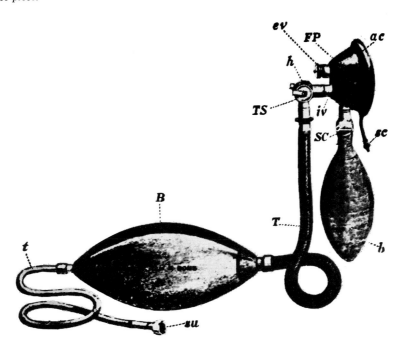

LATER MODEL, *c.* 1890, OF THE TYPE OF NITROUS OXIDE APPARATUS

first put on the market by the firm of Coxeter & Son in August 1868.

available in 1885. A nitrous oxide/oxygen apparatus of their manufacture bears an American patent number referable to this date (the apparatus is in the collection in the Geoffrey Kaye Museum, Melbourne, see p. 133).

In 1883, Paul Bert had recommended a technique using pure nitrous oxide for induction, followed by a mixture of nitrous oxide with oxygen, in the same proportions as in air. A Viennese dentist, H.T.

Hillischer, produced a somewhat cumbersome apparatus in 1886, (Fig. 3.11) which was described by Hewitt as 'unsatisfactory'. Frederick Hewitt himself is a towering figure in these developments, whose apparatus is described in the following pages. Stimulated by his work, S.S.White designed apparatus which was the forerunner of the nitrous oxide/oxygen sequential machines of today. Among those who also produced important innovations

The first to use the two gases in
combination. This fearsome piece
was described by Hewitt as
'portable enough', but he
complained that small alterations of
the oxygen control on the mask
meant considerable alterations to
the percentage. As a result, Hewitt
devised his stopcock. (p. 125.)

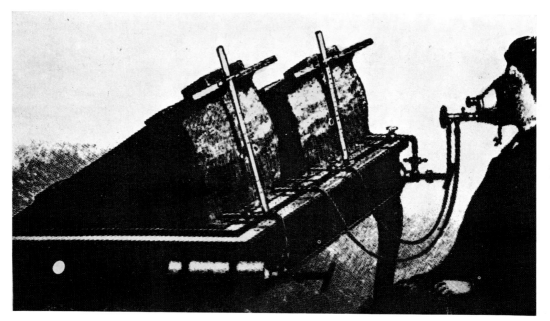

were Frederick Jay Cotton, 1869–1938, of Boston
and Walter M.Boothby, 1880–1953, of Rochester
Minnesota,* who in 1912 were the first to use the
'bubble-bottle' for visible gas measurements in
anaesthesia[22]. This development was taken up by
J.T.Gwathmey and by Marshall, Boyle and others
whose machines are described below.

Earlier apparatus such as that of Charles Teter of
Cleveland, Ohio, also exerted considerable influence,
though this had no measuring device. Teter gave
close instructions as to minute by minute variations
in the oxygen flow to avoid cyanosis while maintaining adequate anaesthesia[23]. At the other extreme,
the secondary saturation technique of McKesson,
while apparently successful in his hands, produced
cyanotic effects which gave many other anaesthetists,
particularly the British, nasty frights. McKesson's
very successful nitrous oxide/oxygen intermittent
flow machine is described in detail below. (CKC 32,
60, p. 155).

Other influential designs were those of Dennis
Jackson, of St Louis, who demonstrated the practical
use of carbon dioxide absorbtion[24]: and the Guy-
Ross (Edinburgh) apparatus in which oxygen was
'injected' by a hand bellows. The Charles King
Collection contains an incomplete specimen of the
latter, presented by Dr H.Jarvis.

Among the important ideas put forward in the
Great War period was that of George W.Crile of

---

* Better known for the B.L.B. oxygen mask (Boothby,
Lovelace, Bulbulian). Boothby was awarded the highest
award in American Aviation, the Collier trophy, for his work
on supplying oxygen to pilots at high altitude.

Cleveland, who invented the term *anoci-association* and whose book of 1914[25] gave a wonderful description of the origins and treatment of shock as then envisaged. The use of nitrous oxide combined with narcotic premedication and local infiltration techniques should have induced a revolution in anaesthesia. As it was, anaesthetists paid much lip-service to the innovation, and continued to pour ether and chloroform on to masks.

Nevertheless the continued use of nitrous oxide and oxygen, augmented by chloroform or ether, only went to prove the safety of 'gas', provided that its limitations were realized. The development of the closed circuit for cyclopropane by Ralph Waters in the 1930's caused but a momentary pause in the use of nitrous oxide, in spite of the enthusiasm of Waters himself and of Nosworthy in this country.

In obstetrics too, the analgesic effects of the gas were made available through Minnitt's apparatus of 1933; this will be more fully described in a later section.

The toxic effects of prolonged administration of nitrous oxide have recently been surveyed by Parbrook[26], but this aspect of the drug has in no way prevented its becoming the anaesthetic in most common use at the present time.

CKC 4: WHITE NITROUS OXIDE BAG, *c.* 1865

The attribution of this bag (Fig. 3.12) to the manufacturing firm of S.S.White,* Philadelphia, was made by Charles King. It is the archetypal apparatus as used in the original days by Gardner Quincy

* See CKC 14, White gas and oxygen apparatus, for biographical details (p. 132).

Colton (and probably by other showmen) and by Horace Wells in 1844.

As has been told, Colton continued his itinerant demonstrations after the Wells fiasco, and when he reintroduced the use of nitrous oxide into dental work in 1862 (see p. 112), it was still with this type of apparatus though of much greater capacity. Shortly after, however, he began to use generators of his own or Sprague's design for the production of the gas from ammonium nitrate, (Figs. 3.13, 3.14) and was able to lead it directly to the patient from the gas-holder. Nevertheless when the idea first crossed the Atlantic and was used in a trial series by Samuel Lee Rymer (Fig. 3.15) at the National Dental Hospital, the latter reverted to the older method (Fig. 3.16). Rymer wrote 'The usual method of inhaling nitrous oxide is from a bladder filled with the gas and to which is attached a tube of wood. The mouthpiece is held by the right hand of the person inhaling the gas, the nostrils being closed by the left. The tube is placed in the mouth and the gas breathed from and into the bladder . . . a vulcanised india-rubber bag and a bladder were alternately used to hold the gas. The tube or mouthpiece was of large aperture to admit of quick inhalation—an all important point where excitement is not wanted'[27].

Rymer recommended that the administration should be under the direction of a professional man, and stated that one person should give the gas, while the extraction was performed by another. Nevertheless he was unconvinced, and the use of nitrous oxide in England was not popularized till Thomas Evans introduced it in 1868.

Rymer's description is exactly that of the present apparatus. The wooden mouth-piece and stopcock are attached to a bag of oiled silk of about 2 litre capacity. In use, air was excluded as far as possible (a nose clip was often provided) and it is apparent

FIG. 3.12. S.S. WHITE NITROUS OXIDE BAG, c. 1865.
Similar to those used by Horace Wells, 1844, Gardner Quincy Colton, 1844–62, and by Samuel Lee Rymer 1863. The bag capacity is approximately two litres. In this example, it is made of oiled silk, but other materials were also used, such as animal bladders.
CKC 4

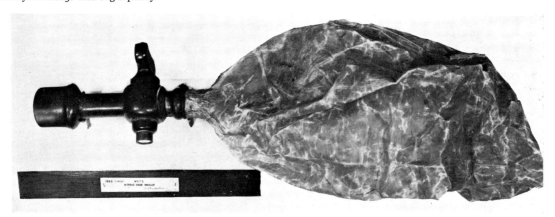

that the size of this bag barely provided enough gas for adequate analgesia. If such a size was in fact used by Wells, then it is likely that herein lay the primary cause of his failure. W.D.A.Smith has recently conducted personal experiments using a similar bag; he records that rebreathing till cyanosis occurred did not produce unconsciousness[28]. Colton and Evans, in 1868, were using bags of thirty litre capacity. In any event, with the re-introduction, English anaesthetists and dental surgeons such as Clover and Coleman very quickly began to devise other and more complicated methods of administration.

In 1870, the S.S.White Company of Philadelphia, following the lead of Coxeter of London, introduced a surgeon's case containing a mouth-piece and bag, with a cylinder of nitrous oxide. Thus these two firms were the first to introduce the liquefaction and distribution of nitrous oxide[29].

FIG. 3.13. SPRAGUE NITROUS
OXIDE GENERATOR, *c.* 1863.
The controlled heating of
ammonium nitrate produces the
gas, which is passed through wash-
bottles containing ferrous sulphate
and water, one of which contained a
stick of caustic potash, for the
removal of chlorine. The gas was
passed direct from the gas-holder to
the patient. (See Fig. 3.9).
From Turnbull,L. (1896).
Artificial Anaesthesia. Philadelphia.
p. 245

IG. 3.14. S.S.WHITE NITROUS
OXIDE GENERATOR, 1867.
H is the mouth-piece, shown in
detail in Figs. 4 and 5, one way
valves being arranged as at R and S.
From S.S.White, (1867) *Catalogue
of Dental Materials.* p. 143.

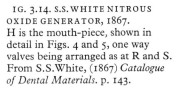

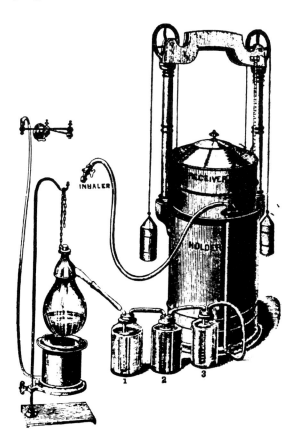

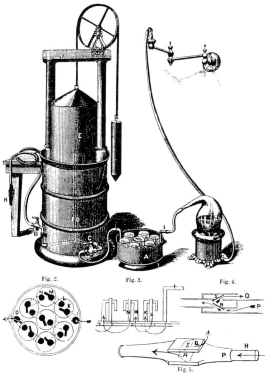

FIG. 3.15. SAMUEL LEE RYMER,
1833–1909,
who used nitrous oxide at the
National Dental Hospital in
1863.[27] His results were not
satisfactory.
From 1856 onwards Rymer was
greatly involved, with John Tomes
and others, in the reform of the
dental profession.
Photograph from obituary notice,
British Dental Journal. (1909) **30**, i,
282

FIG. 3.16. SAMUEL RYMER'S
METHOD OF ADMINISTERING
NITROUS OXIDE, 1863,
Similar to that of Horace Wells in
1844.
From Rottenstein, J.B. (1880)
Traité d'anésthèsie chirurgicale.
Paris, p. 150 (In Duncum, 1947.)

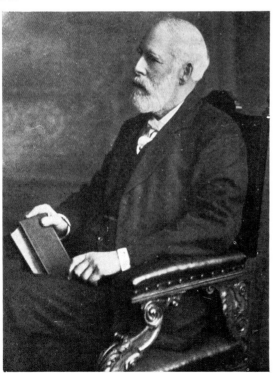

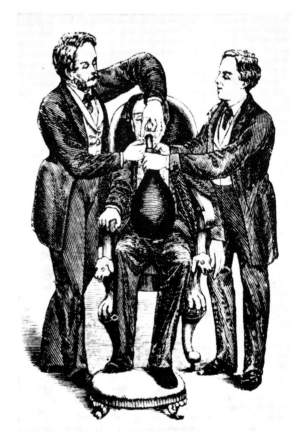

CKC 7: CLOVER NITROUS OXIDE-ETHER APPARATUS 1876

Joseph Clover produced this ingenious piece in 1876, one year before his Portable Regulating Ether Inhaler (see p. 14), and he himself declared he preferred it to the latter. Clover worked upon its development for several years and different forms existed, of which the Charles King specimen (Fig. 3.17) appears to be a late type, particularly in possessing twin cylinders, a feature which has not been found in any of the early drawings or descriptions (but compare the 1914 drawing, Fig. 3.18). When Clover first described it in 1876[30], he stated that he had used it on some two thousand three hundred patients at St Bartholomew's, University College, St Mary's and the Dental Hospitals.

The apparatus consists essentially of a gas cylinder, and an ether vessel with a Cattlin bag and face piece (Figs. 3.17, 3.18). The bag was described by W.A.N.Cattlin, dentist, of Brighton, and was mentioned by Clover in 1868; the name was thereafter commonly used for all rebreathing bags. Clover says it was 15 in long and contained 400 in (*sic*) i.e. about 6 litres. The Collection specimen is not so large, but cannot be measured, as the rubber has hardened. Through the bag Clover passed a rubber tube connecting the regulator on the face piece to the outlet of the nitrous oxide control tube (Figs. 3.19, 3.20). This control tube closely resembled that of the Clover ether apparatus (Fig. 3.21 cf. Fig. 1.11), and allowed the admission of air or nitrous oxide to the bag, or, if the ether vaporizer control was 'on', a mixture of gas and ether. Air was not admitted till cyanosis or jactitation occurred and as late as 1914, Buxton, enthusiastically describing this apparatus, wrote 'slight cyanosis and breath holding are not necessarily signs for admitting air. If the face-piece

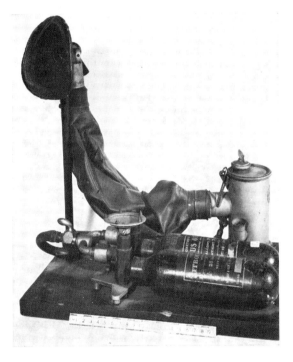

FIG. 3.17. CLOVER NITROUS OXIDE/ETHER APPARATUS, 1876. As the first attempt to use a gas/ether sequence, this ingenious apparatus was an important step in the long progress towards safer and more certain anaesthesia. CKC 7

is lifted too soon the patient will rapidly 'come-out' of the nitrous oxide narcosis, and his blood not being sufficiently saturated with ether, he will commence to struggle. On the other hand, if the ventilation of the lungs by air is delayed too long, respiration will be seriously impeded and the heart become embarrassed. One, if not more deaths have occurred through this accident, although the watchful administrator can hardly overlook the obvious signs of danger, such as failure of respiration associated with deep cyanosis'[31].

FIG. 3.18. CLOVER SEQUENTIAL
APPARATUS,
to show large-bore tube extended
through the Cattlin bag. Ether and
nitrous oxide controls may be seen
on the ether container, and
mixture control on the angle-piece.
The mask has an expiratory valve.
The ether container was hung from
the lapel.
From Buxton,D.W. (1914)
Anaesthetics. London: Lewis. p. 170

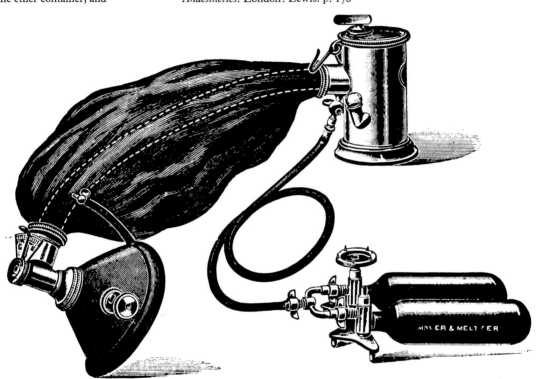

One cannot but admire the skill and nerve with which Clover and the other 'watchful administrators' undertook anaesthesia under such conditions; conditions quite unacceptable to the modern anaesthetist.

Buxton suggested opening the gas inlet, after detaching the tube, in order that the patient may draw in some air, once ether anaesthesia is established. He also said 'when, owing to respiratory spasm, or persistent cyanosis, oxygen seems indicated, it can be admitted through this tap.' Having made such a positive suggestion regarding the use of oxygen, it is curious that Buxton did not consider it as an essential, though he was writing some thirty years after Clover, and after Paul Bert's (1878) work on gaseous partial pressures. Furthermore, compressed oxygen had been available since 1889, when Hewitt introduced his nitrous oxide/oxygen apparatus. In 1968, the Clover sequential apparatus was discussed in detail by Nunn[32].

The Clover 'Combined nitrous oxide and ether' apparatus was the first practical method for the sequential use of anaesthetic vapours. As such, it was a notable landmark in the development of anaesthetic apparatus.

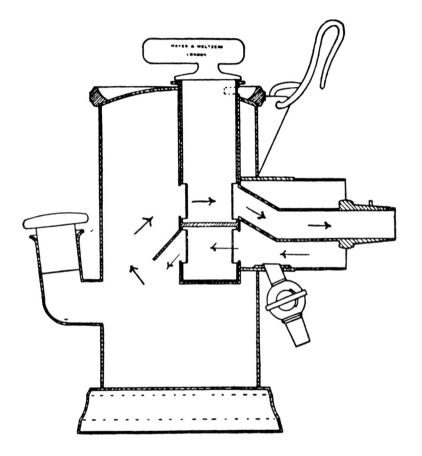

FIG. 3.19. THE CLOVER ETHER CHAMBER IN SECTION.
The arrows demonstrate flow of gas through the container when in the 'ether on' position. Rotation of the top tap allowed the inhalation of nitrous oxide alone. Ether with air could be administered by removing the nitrous oxide tubing, but the inlet for air was then of a size which would be considered well below safe levels by modern standards.
It will be seen that the control tube bears a close resemblance to that which Clover used in his portable ether inhaler (Fig. 3.21 and Fig. 1.11)
From Buxton,D.W. (1914) *op. cit.* p. 171

FIG. 3.20. BUXTON'S MODIFIED
AND IMPROVED ETHER INHALER.
The improvement consisted in
making the parts easily separable,
as shown, in order to facilitate
cleaning. The tube shown above the
bag passes through it, to yoke with
the ether chamber at one end, and
with the face piece mount at the
other.
From Buxton, D.W. (1914). *op. cit.*
p. 172

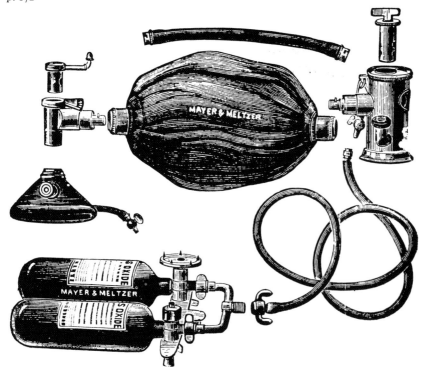

CKC 12: HEWITT NITROUS OXIDE/ OXYGEN STOPCOCK 1893

Twenty-five years after the re-introduction of nitrous oxide, Frederick Hewitt (see Fig. 1.21) was to write: 'cyanosis, jerky and irregular breathing, deep stertor, and clonic movements of the extremities, are symptoms which for many reasons might be dispensed with during the use of nitrous oxide'[33], thus giving the picture of what was considered to be acceptable anaesthesia in 1893. From 1885 onward, however, Hewitt had been experimenting with the use of nitrous oxide, at first alone, then mixed with air, and later with oxygen. As a research worker in this field he was familiar with the writings of Paul Bert[34], who in 1879 had provided satisfactory anaesthesia with his famous nitrous oxide/oxygen pressure chamber: with those of Hillischer[35], a Viennese dentist, who from 1886 had experimented with apparatus providing nitrous oxide and oxygen under atmospheric pressure (see Fig. 3.11); Hillischer proposed the name 'Schlafgas' for the mixture, from the sleep like state produced; he had used it in some 15,000 cases: Hewitt also quoted the work of Witzel[36] of Essen, and H.C.Wood[37] of Philadelphia, both of whom administered nitrous oxide and oxygen. He also mentioned a 'remarkable experiment of M. Claude Martin of Lyons who administered to a dog a mixture of nitrous oxide with 15 per cent oxygen for three consecutive days'.

Hewitt wrote 'In 1886, at the Dental Hospital of London, I commenced a series of experimental administrations of nitrous oxide and oxygen, at ordinary atmospheric pressures . . . no less than thirteen distinct plans were tried, each of which necessitated a different form of apparatus'[38].

The present piece of apparatus (Fig. 3.22) is the ultimate in this series, described by Hewitt both in

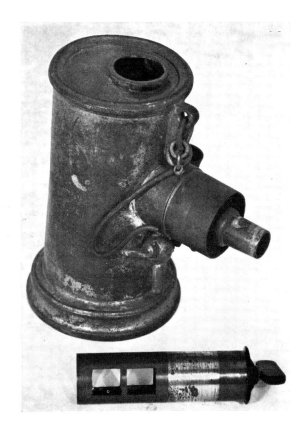

FIG. 3.21. ETHER CONTROL, CLOVER SEQUENTIAL APPARATUS, 1876.
The resemblance to that in the ether inhaler of 1877 is notable. (see fig. 1.11). The central tube from the canister passes nitrous oxide or ether to the mask. The larger outer tube returns expired vapours from the bag. The nitrous oxide inlet (with tap) may also be used for air. Its small size will be noted.

FIG. 3.22. HEWITT NITROUS
OXIDE/OXYGEN STOPCOCK, 1893.
CKC 12

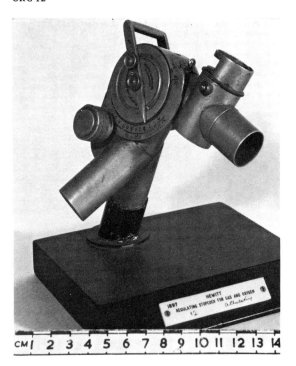

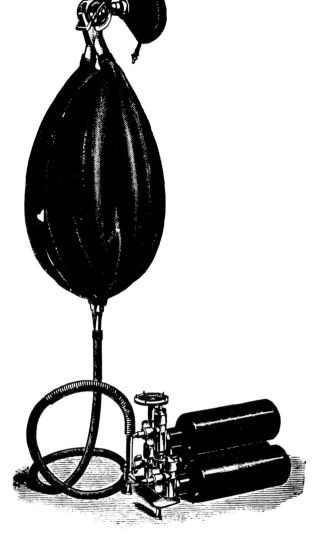

FIG. 3.23. Hewitt stopcock as used
with double reservoir bag and bank
of three cylinders, the upper one
containing oxygen. (See Fig. 3.24
for detail of the double yoke and
tube.
From Hewitt,F.W. (1897).
*Administration of Nitrous Oxide and
Oxygen.* p. 24

his book of 1897[38], and in a paper to the British Dental Association in 1894[39], though not in his book of 1893[33] where an earlier type is shown; both patterns were described by Barbara Duncum in 1947[40]. The later model was therefore developed in 1893 and 1894, before the date given by Charles King, who suggested 1897; it does not seem subsequently to have received the attention it deserves.

Hewitt gave a detailed survey of the use of mixtures of nitrous oxide and oxygen in gasometers, in fixed proportions, stating that 5–8 per cent served him best. He warned against keeping the mixture for too long, stating that Ludwig had found traces of the higher oxides of nitrogen at the end of a week. He found however that a regulating apparatus was really necessary, and so developed the present form.

In enumerating eleven requirements, Hewitt stated, among other needs:

1 There must be a plentiful supply of the two gases from easily and quietly working cylinders.
2 The bags into which the gases pass must be capable of being kept partly and equally distended during the administration.
3 The bags must be as close as possible to the face piece:
4 The channels throughout the apparatus must be sufficiently large to avoid any stress whatever being thrown upon the circulation;
5 The regulating portion of the apparatus must allow of very small increments and decrements in the proportion of oxygen breathed:
6 There must be accurately working valves: (a) for preventing all re-breathing and (b) for preventing diffusion between the contents of one bag and the other.

The apparatus as fully designed by Hewitt, is shown in Fig. 3.23, which is taken from his book of 1897. The regulator is identical with the Charles King specimen and other points are the double india-rubber tubes (one inside the other), the double cylinder union (Fig. 3.24) and the two bags joined by a common septum (Fig. 3.25).

The regulator is shown in exploded form in Fig. 3.26; the oxygen chamber, OC, communicates with the larger nitrous oxide chamber through ten small holes (three only appear in the figure, marked OO). AH is the air hole, fully exposed when the control lever is moved to the 'air' position. PD is a 'partial diaphragm' designed to deflect the exhaled gas towards the expiratory valve. The rotating inner mixture chamber, shown separately, has a long slot, S. Its rotation by the control lever causes the exposure of the various ports, that is, a number of the ten oxygen holes are uncovered, and mixing occurs.

Hewitt wrote 'It may thus be said that directly the indicator is made to point to 'N$_2$O', there passes through the stopcock a continuous and large stream of nitrous oxide. And that any number of small streams of oxygen, from one to ten inclusive may, at will, be added to this continuous stream of nitrous oxide.' The oxygen control, through which these 'small streams' pass, corresponds to the 'gauge-plate' of the S.S.White gas and oxygen apparatus (see p. 133).

Nevertheless, he added that it was impossible to state, with precision, what percentage of oxygen will come through at any given setting, for one apparatus will be found to differ slightly from another and much will depend upon the relative sizes of the bags at that moment.

Hewitt devoted a whole chapter to the minutiae of administering the gases, all of it sound anaesthetic practice, referring to posture, noise, dental props, (of which his own design was by far the most satisfactory) and to the signs of anaesthesia as

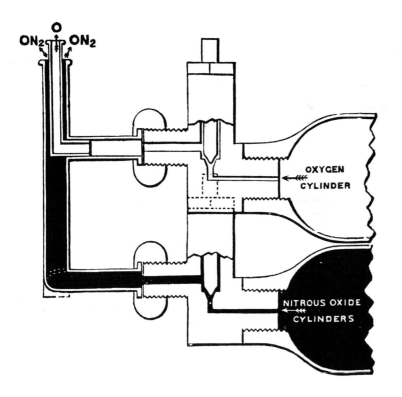

ON₂ O ON₂

FIG. 3.24. DOUBLE CYLINDER YOKE
with large-bore nitrous oxide tube, through which the smaller oxygen tube passes to the bag.
From Hewitt, F.W. (1897). *op. cit.*, p. 26

OXYGEN CYLINDER

NITROUS OXIDE CYLINDERS

FIG. 3.25. HEWITT MAY HAVE ATTEMPTED TO EQUALIZE THE PRESSURE

in the two bags by arranging a conjoined pair joined by a common septum. There is no mention in this book, or in Hewitt's other writings, that this was his specific intention, but he did regard equal distension as important. The entry of the double gas tube is shown.
From Hewitt, F.W. (1897). *op. cit.* p. 27

FIG. 3.26. HEWITT STOPCOCK IN EXPLODED FORM.
(See text).
From Hewitt, F.W. (1897). *op. cit.* p. 29

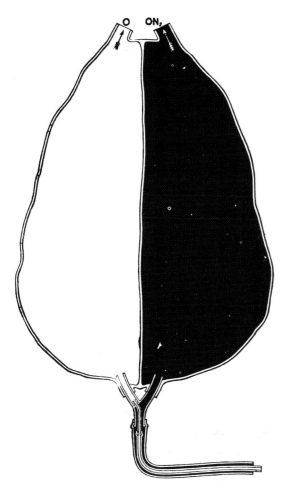

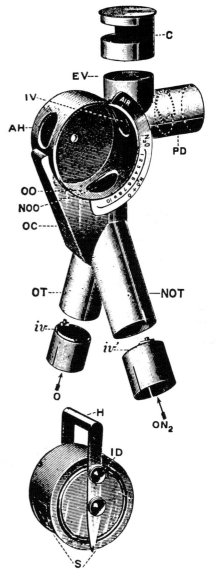

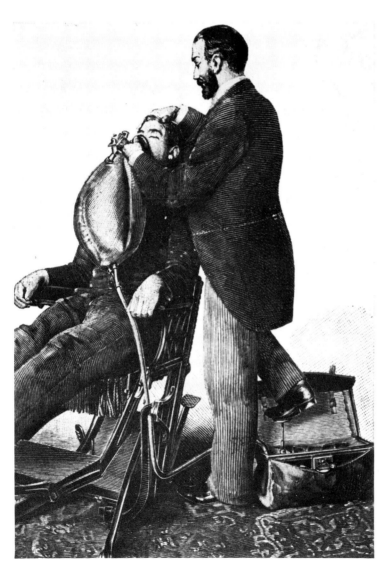

FIG. 3.27. ADMINISTRATION OF
NITROUS OXIDE AND OXYGEN
with Hewitt's apparatus.
From Hewitt,F.W. (1897). *op. cit.*
p. 44

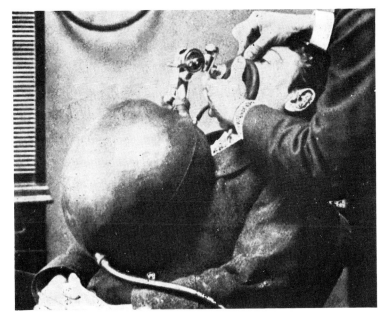

FIG. 3.28. DETAIL OF USE OF
SINGLE DIVIDED BAG AND
HEWITT'S STOPCOCK.
From Bellamy Gardner, H. (1916).
Manual of Surgical Anaesthesia.
p. 102

modified by varying percentages of oxygen. (Figs. 3.27, 3.28). It is of interest, however, that he made no attempt to continue the anaesthesia during the operation, which was usually for dental extractions. He stated that the duration of inhalation necessary was on average 110 seconds, 'i.e. nearly twice the length of the average nitrous oxide inhalation' (without oxygen), and he remarked that it was not easy to judge the point at which the face mask was to be removed and the operation begun. The average duration of the available anaesthesia was a mere forty-four seconds, though this could be extended to sixty or seventy seconds by lengthening the administration of the gases to some three minutes. 'In the event of unexpected difficulties arising in the operation, the anaesthetist is rightly expected to give

the signal for discontinuing the extraction'[41]. Hewitt did not recommend reapplying the face piece in these circumstances, preferring to allow the patient to recover, to wash out his mouth and to be re-anaesthetized!

Nasal administration was found to be difficult, owing to variations in bag pressure.

Though others preceded him in the use of oxygen with nitrous oxide, it was undoubtedly Hewitt's work which finally demonstrated its value: but in spite of this, the Hewitt double stopcock does not seem to have been popular. It was described again by Hewitt himself in his little book of 1897[38], and by Boyle in 1907[42], by Dudley Buxton[43], and by Bellamy Gardner[44], among others, but these authors also described his simple nitrous oxide/*air* stopcock, and the latter was in use in the casualty department of one of Hewitt's hospitals, as late as 1939. Others modified the apparatus, notably Goodman Levy, who made nasal administration of nitrous oxide–oxygen mixtures more satisfactory by placing the oxygen bag within that for the nitrous oxide. The resulting gas pressures were thus identical, and it was therefore possible to vary the oxygen percentage administered through a nose piece. Previously the necessary excess of pressure needed was found to disturb excessively the proportion of oxygen in the mixture (see Bellamy Gardner)[44].

In addition to those works quoted, the following are the more important papers by Hewitt on the use of oxygen with nitrous oxide:
Lancet, 1889, **i**, 832. On the Anaesthesia produced by the Administration of mixtures of Nitrous Oxide and Oxygen.
Transactions of the Odontological Society of London. 1892. **24**n.s. 194–244.
On the Anaesthetic Effects of Nitrous Oxide when administered with oxygen at ordinary atmospheric pressures, with remarks on 800 cases.

CKC 14: S.S. WHITE GAS AND OXYGEN APPARATUS, *c* 1910

Samuel Stockton White, 1822–1879 (Fig. 3.29), founded the Dental Manufacturing Company, which still bears his name, in 1844. White came of an old New England family, while the Stockton side numbered one who had signed the Declaration of Independence[45]. At the age of sixteen White took up indentures with his uncle, Samuel Wesley Stockton, a pioneer tooth manufacturer in Philadelphia, 'to learn the Art, Trade and Mystery of

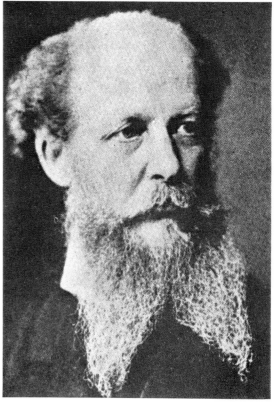

FIG. 3.29. SAMUEL STOCKTON WHITE, 1822–1879, founder of the Dental Manufacturing Company in 1844. See White's nitrous oxide bag, 1865 (p. 117). (CKC 4) and White's gas/oxygen apparatus, *c.* 1910. (CKC 14) From Archer, W.H. (1944) Historical Sketch of Anaesthesia. *Curr. Res. Anesth. Analg.* **23**. 244

Manufacturing Teeth' 'and after the manner of an apprentice to serve the said Samuel Stockton . . . the full term of five years.'; the master agreed to give instruction in the art of dentistry and the boy was also taught by a well known dental surgeon, Dr Haven White, who was not a relative. On qualifying in 1843, the young Samuel began the practice of dentistry with his uncle, and undertook to superintend the manufacturing processes. He was so successful in this that in 1844 he began his own

FIG. 3.30. CONTROLS AND
'GAUGE-PLATE'
of the S.S. White Nitrous oxide/
oxygen apparatus in Geoffrey Kaye
Museum, Melbourne. The nitrous
oxide control (lower right) is to be
fully opened after opening the
cylinder controls (at back). The
oxygen control (highest knob)
admits oxygen to a degree indicated
on the semi-circular 'gauge-plate'.

S.S.White's pamphlet of 1903,[46]
states 'exact and predetermined
percentages are neither practical nor
desirable.' The mixing chamber is
central and a wide-bore tube led to
the face mask. This model bears an
American patent date, October 12,
1885, which appears to be earlier
than White's production of oxygen
cylinders (the accepted date for
which is 1888).

business in a garret, assisted by his younger brother, James William, who later achieved a reputation as the Editor of *Dental Cosmos*. S.S.White was a master mould cutter, carving the moulds himself and making the final models with his own hands. Business prospered and the firm branched out into the manufacture of all types of dental equipment.

In 1870, the firm introduced liquified nitrous oxide in cylinders (see p. 113) and began the development of apparatus for its use. In 1888, the Company commenced the manufacture of compressed oxygen for therapeutic use, following demands by doctors for a convenient method of delivery of oxygen. The Company was diffident about it, as is shown by a note in one of its files, 'the use of oxygen is new, and its value as a remedial agent unsettled; there is even a possibility that its employment is a mere fad which when it has run its brief day of popularity will vanish into the limbo of buried hopes.'

In the 1890's, the S.S.White Company produced the first apparatus for anaesthesia by the 'non-asphyxial' method of Hewitt. This was indeed a pioneer development, being among the earliest to use a modern yoke system for the mixing and delivery of the gases. The specimen in the Charles King Collection is an example of this series. King himself attributed it to this same period (1899). The White apparatus in its early development carried either two or three cylinders, whereas the King example is a four cylinder machine with two double yokes. A catalogue of S.S.White of 1903 shows both two and three cylinder models, the latter costing fifty dollars, without cylinders. The oxygen cylinders were painted red, those for nitrous oxide being black, and the gases were led to the two-gallon bags, each with its own control, which passed them to a mixing chamber, and thence via a wide bore tube to the face mask. In the 1903 model no reduction in

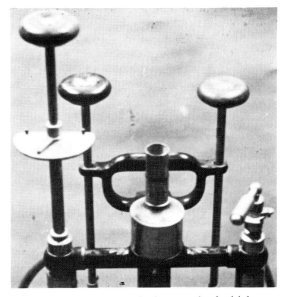

pressure was available. The 'gauge-plate' which controlled the oxygen was described as 'especially designed to enable the operator to follow Dr Hewitt's method, the valve opening enlarging regularly as the handle is turned. It must be understood however that exact and predetermined percentages are neither practical nor desirable'[46]. A two cylinder specimen of this type exists in the Geoffrey Kaye Museum, Melbourne (Fig. 3.30). It bears the very early U.S. patent date, October 12, 1885, but it is thought that this cannot refer to the oxygen side of the apparatus, since S.S.White did not produce oxygen cylinders until 1888, while the Hewitt gauge-plate, which is a feature of this early pattern, was not described till 1893 (see p. 127).

The Charles King specimen (Fig. 3.31) has achieved a greater degree of sophistication. A recognizably modern stand (though without wheels)

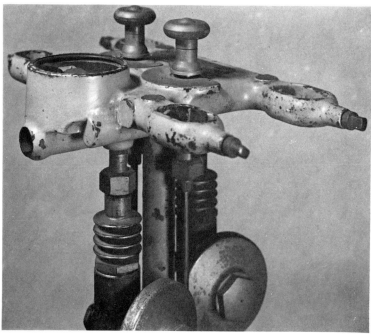

FIG. 3.31. S.S. WHITE NITROUS OXIDE/OXYGEN APPARATUS *c.* 1910.
Showing a double-yoked head for four cylinders, the reducing valves (see Fig. 3.32) and the two rotating mixture controls. The glass dome over mixing chamber is missing. The gases passed to the patient through the wide-bore opening below. There were no reservoir bags.
CKC 14

carries a double-yoked head for the four cylinders. Copper tubes lead the gases to quite elegant and efficient looking reducing valves, and thence to two controls, each rotating through a half circle, and marked 0–10 for both oxygen and nitrous oxide. The mixing chamber has a curious valve arrangement with two moving aluminium flaps, the function of which has not been determined. The reducing valves consist of a tube turned in steel (Figs. 3.32, 3.33) with a spring and flexible brass diaphragm carried in a side drum, the former by its resistance controlling the flow of gas through a brass toggle device. The spring has no screw control, but a safety-valve is provided. Further control of the flow is produced by a steel pin, and by a very tight pack-

ing of wool (40cm of wool of about 1cm diameter being packed into 2.5cm of the steel tube) held in place by copper gauze filters. Flanges on the main tube are designed to provide a large area at ambient temperature, and so prevent freezing.

This model is not dated, but it carries a 'patent pending' label, on which it is described as 'apparatus No. 3, Serial No. 18, made in U.S.A.' by 'the S.S. White Dental Mfg.Co.' The date of 1899 given by Charles King is probably too early and an amended date of *circa* 1910 is suggested.

FIG. 3.32. REDUCING VALVE
of S.S.White apparatus. (See
Figs 3.31 and 3.33).

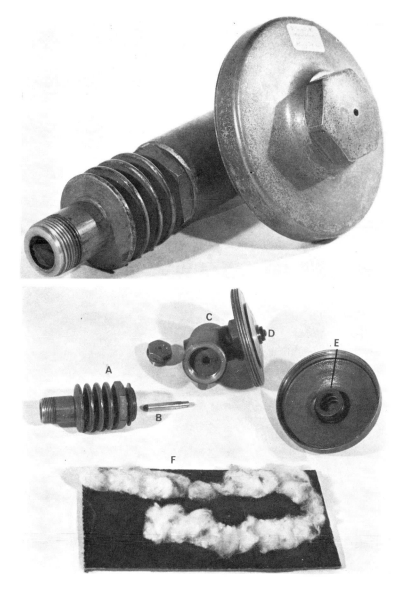

FIG. 3.33. REDUCING VALVE IN
EXPLODED STATE.
In spite of its age the craftsmanship
was such that this valve was readily
dismantled to show A, a heavy
flanged tube carrying pin B which
engages with a toggle inside tube C.
This in turn moves the mechanism
consisting of a brass diaphragm D,
working against a strong spring E.
The lower end of the flanged tube A
was packed very tightly with about
40cm of 1cm diameter wool (F).
Also shown separated is the nut
carrying a safety-valve.

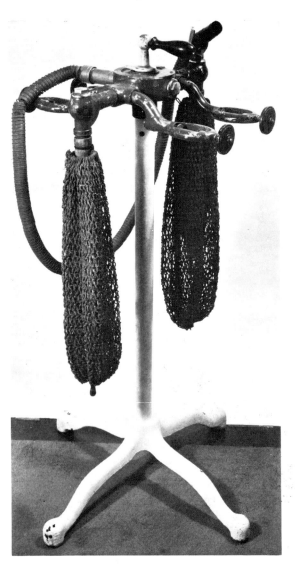

CKC 15: CLARK NITROUS OXIDE/OXYGEN APPARATUS *c.* 1910

This apparatus resembles the S.S.White (No. 14) and was also attributed by Charles King to the year 1899. It was made by the A.C.Clark Co. of Chicago and is described in a pamphlet as '*The Clark New Model Gas Apparatus for excavating dentine, the removal of pulps etc.*' This pamphlet is marked '1915'[47], and a photograph shows a machine identical to the King specimen, sold at a price of seventy-five dollars. It is described as a 'simple apparatus for the administration of N_2O or Oxy. pure or both combined in any desired proportions. The gases are thoroughly mixed in an efficient mixing chamber and controlled by one handle. This outfit is built for the purpose of administering the two gases for analgesia or anaesthesia. Previous Clark outfits were mainly for administering N_2O only . . . these two gases in combination make the most perfect anaesthetic that has ever been invented. A small amount of nitrous oxid (sic), in combination with oxygen, can be administered and in almost every case an analgesic anaesthesia produced. In this condition the patient is awake to all of the senses except pain . . . and he can readily be kept in this condition for almost any length of time desired, without any danger and without any inconvenience.'

The apparatus consists of two double cylinder yokes mounted on a four-footed stand (Fig. 3.34). No reducing valves are provided, the gases going direct to a mixing chamber built into the casting. The oxygen yokes are painted red, and the nitrous oxide black; each has a reservoir bag of about 4 gallons (18 litres), in a string expander. On top of the mixing chamber a control handle moves through a half-circle, painted segments indicating the mixture from 100 per cent oxygen to 100 per cent

FIG. 3.35. JAY A. HEIDBRINK,
1875–1957.
From *American Dental Science
Annual*, (1957) p. 45

nitrous oxide. The wide-bore tubing is wire reinforced and the face and nasal masks have an inspiratory (air) inlet and expiratory valves. The apparatus was described by King himself [48, 49].

The absence of reducing valves, with the consequence surging and absence of pressure control, together with the probability of freezing of the cylinder valves must have made 'analgesic anaesthesia' rather more difficult to achieve than the glowing eulogy of the advertisers pamphlet would suggest. Nevertheless the S.S.White and Clark machines represented an important step in the development of apparatus for the delivery of combined gases. Upon consideration, the date of 1899 given by Charles King must be too early. Like the S.S.White apparatus, the Clark represents developments taking place in the first decade of the new century and should be ascribed to *c*. 1910.

CKC 22: HEIDBRINK NITROUS OXIDE/OXYGEN APPARATUS *c*. 1920

Jay Albion Heidbrink, 1875–1957 (Fig. 3.35), of Minneapolis, became a distinguished anaesthetist who had set up in dental practice in Wisconsin, in about 1890. His 'Memoirs'[50] describe his early adventures using cocaine, alcohol (locally) and gas supplied from a bag, much as Colton had done forty years before. But though his descriptions make amusing reading—'he got out of the chair and attacked! I threw him on the floor and sat on him for a while'—Heidbrink was dissatisfied with such methods, and when in 1903 Charles Teter of Cleveland showed him a gas/oxygen machine, he immediately bought one. Finding drawbacks to the Teter apparatus, he redesigned it. 'Pressure in the

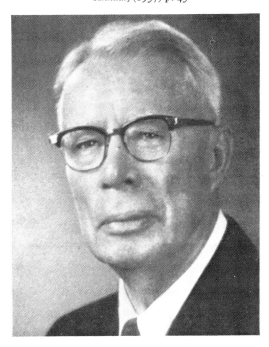

bags was never constant', he wrote 'I positioned these bags, one on top of the other, on a platform . . . and superimposed a weight to equalise the pressures. The valves were slotted to provide finer control. A third bag—a rebreathing bag—was interposed between the mixing bag and the tubing to the inhaler. At that time, because of moisture in the gas, the opening from the tank would sometimes freeze. . . . An electric light bulb placed in the mixing chamber prevented this and warmed the gases'[51]. Heidbrink found the remodelled apparatus was better, but still not good enough, so he designed his own.

Here he produced his stroke of genius. In his own words 'I described a valve to one of the mechanics

FIG. 3.36. HEIDBRINK
'ANESTHETIZER'.
From Gwathmey, J.T. (1925)
Anesthesia. New York: Macmillan.
p. 148
Identical with the King Collection
specimen but for the stopwatch.
Note the control working over a
gauge-plate marked 'FORCE'.

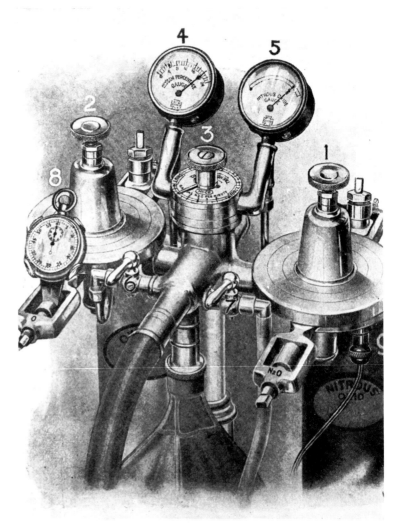

which would reduce tank pressures to working pressures. When he informed me that such valves were already available, I purchased two'[51]. The success of this machine was such that the Dean of the Minnesota University Dental School and the local dentists asked Heidbrink to make models for their use. His first commercial machine was produced in 1912 and cost thirty-two dollars. Later Heidbrink was joined by a salesman, Walter McGillivra, who sold many machines and who became an accomplished anaesthetist, being in charge of anaesthesia at Harvard University Dental School.

The date of 1912 is noteworthy, for the Heidbrink machine of this date became his 'Model A'. Twenty models then appeared, the latest being 'Model T', which gave way in 1938 to his Simplex Dental Model. This remained in use for many years. The Charles King Collection no. 22 has no series letter, but bears the individual number 1246. Charles King himself dated it from 1910, but it is now thought that this date is somewhat early. The 1925 edition of Gwathmey's text-book has a picture and description of an identical model (Fig. 3.36), whereas it is not mentioned in the first edition of 1914, in spite of the comprehensive nature of this book. It would therefore appear to be midway in the Heidbrink series, dating from about 1920.

The specimen has yokes for four cylinders with two flat reducing valves, one for each pair; an oxygen percentage gauge is marked to 24 per cent, (arrowed at 20 per cent) and a nitrous oxide dial is arrowed but not numbered (Figs. 3.36, 3.37). The mixing chamber has a control knob working over a gauge-plate, marked 'FORCE' and divided into forty equal unnumbered divisions which represent a maximum of twenty gallons of nitrous oxide per minute. The model shown by Gwathmey has a stopwatch

(mounted in one of the oxygen yokes). Heidbrink regarded this as an important item for training purposes. He wrote 'I found . . . that beginners readily became fairly competent anaesthetists when given a definite procedure to follow. Of course, all continued to learn from experience. . . .' 'In the beginning the trainee was permitted only to keep the inhaler firmly in place at all times, in order to aquaint him with its importance. Then he was allowed to manipulate the gas machine. If he made mistakes, I immediately made the correction. If he repeated the error, I would give him a light kick on the shin and repeat with progressively harder ones till he discovered and corrected the error'[52].

CKC 24: GWATHMEY NITROUS OXIDE, OXYGEN, ETHER APPARATUS 1915

James Tayloe Gwathmey (Fig. 3.38) was born in Norfolk, Virginia, 10 September 1863, and died in Arkansas on 11 February 1944. He became consulting anaesthetist to the Metropolitan and other New York hospitals, early in this century, and was one of the first physicians in the United States to confine himself entirely to anaesthetic practice[53]. Gwathmey was well known for his advocacy of oil-ether rectal anesthesia, on which he read his first papers in 1913[54, 55]. Faulconer and Keys state that by 1930 he was able to report 20,000 successful cases of the use of rectal ether in midwifery. In 1914, collaborating with Charles Baskerville, Professor of Chemistry at City of New York College, Gwathmey published his comprehensive textbook, *Anesthesia*, with a second edition in 1925, an important work in the development of anaesthesia in America. In 1913,

FIG. 3.37. HEIDBRINK NITROUS
OXIDE/OXYGEN APPARATUS.
CKC 22

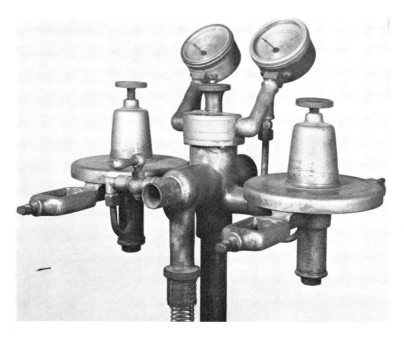

as President of the New York Society of Anesthetists, Gwathmey was largely instrumental in
incorporating that society as the American Association, now the American Society of Anesthesiologists. As a serving officer in the First World War,
Gwathmey was an anaesthetist to the American Red
Cross Hospital in France. Here he renewed acquaintance with H.E.G.Boyle, of St Bartholomew's
Hospital, who used Gwathmey's ideas in the
development of his own apparatus. (see p. 146). In
a paper on anaesthesia for military surgery, Boyle
wrote in 1917, 'my own interest in the matter is due
entirely to Dr James T.Gwathmey of New York,
whom I met at the Congress in 1912. He persuaded

me to get a machine and try for myself, and I have
not regretted it. Gwathmey is one of the greatest
authorities on anaesthesia in the United States, and
it has been my privilege and pleasure to have him by
me whilst I have been working at the 1st London
General Hospital'[56].

Gwathmey himself had been greatly influenced by
the papers and work of Dennis Jackson[57], of
Willis Gatch and especially of Frederick Jay Cotton,
1869–1938, and Walter Boothby, 1880–1953, who,
working at Harvard in the first decade of the century,
described the principles and practice of nitrous
oxide-oxygen apparatus culminating in their perfected apparatus of 1912[58]. Gatch had also pro-

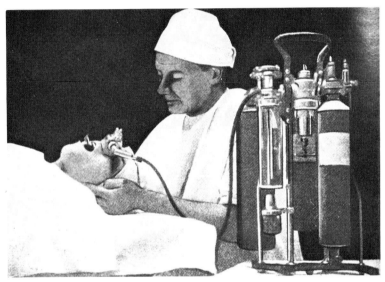

FIG. 3.38. JAMES TAYLOE
GWATHMEY, 1863–1944.
Gwathmey administering nitrous
oxide/oxygen from his own
apparatus. Note the mixing
chamber, the heated water-sight
feed bottle and the carrying handle.
Two cylinders of nitrous oxide and
one of oxygen were coupled.
From Gwathmey, J.T. (1914)
Anesthesia. New York: Appleton.
p. 174

duced his nitrous oxide/oxygen apparatus at about the same time; his method allowed of rebreathing till slight cyanosis occurred, when oxygen was admitted, a plan reminiscent of the later McKesson. Mention should also be made of the apparatus (*c.* 1900) of Charles Teter of Cleveland, Ohio, which Gwathmey considered to be one of the best then developed. None of these, except that of Cotton and Boothby, had any means of assessing the quantities of gases delivered. With these antecedents, Gwathmey himself introduced his own apparatus in 1912, borrowing a device which Cotton and Boothby thought of prime importance, namely a method of rendering the flow of gases 'visible so that their proportions may be approximately estimated at a glance'[58]. The specimen in the Charles King Collection (No. 24. Fig. 3.39) was dated to *circa* 1915 by Charles King. It has yokes for two nitrous oxide and one oxygen cylinder, controlled by a simple needle-valve; no pressure reduction system is provided: the gases are led by external tubing to the cap of the water-sight feed bottle, and each 'bubble-tube' has five holes. Gwathmey says that 'the sightfeed enables the anaesthetist to regulate the proportions of the gases very carefully'[59]. In the absence of pressure reduction, this statement seems optimistic. Later examples however, incorporate . . . 'an efficient reducer of small dimensions and light weight' which may have improved the accuracy by a small amount (Fig. 3.39). Other features of the Gwathmey apparatus are a carrying handle and a metal gauze cylinder beneath the nitrous oxide valve, into which a small alcohol lamp was clipped in order to prevent freezing of the valve. Later models also placed a lamp under the water bottle in order to provide a warmed vapour, one of the fallacies of the period (see Fig. 3.39 and p. 45). The Gwathmey apparatus soon developed into a

FIG. 3.39. HEAD OF GWATHMEY
APPARATUS.

Probably an earlier model than that
shown in Fig. 3.38. There is no
reducing valve, the gases passing
direct to the water-sight bottle. The
wire-gauge tube beneath the nitrous
oxide control would hold a candle
or lamp to prevent freezing. The
water bottle may also have been

warmed, as it was thought that
warmed gases assisted the patient.
Gwathmey also insisted on a special
air-tight face mask, with a rubber
facial cuff, and used a 'sliding cuff'
inspiratory and expiratory valve
which allowed regulation of the
degree of rebreathing.
CKC 24

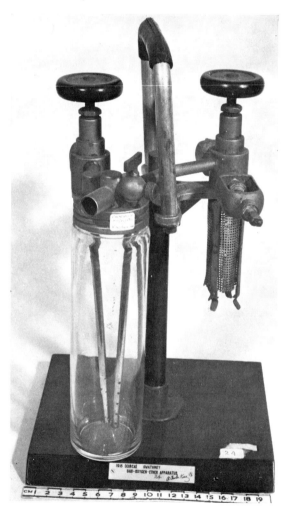

three bottle version for chloroform and ether. To
Cotton and Boothby, and to Gwathmey must be
given the credit of introducing the sight-feed
method into anaesthesia: the early water-bottles
were later supplanted by the dry-bobbin flowmeter,
though it is uncertain whether one actually influenced the other. Equivalent developments were
taking place on the 'industrial' gas front in the same
period, and the priorities would be extremely
difficult to determine. A good account, with many
diagrams, of the development of flowmeters, is
given by Geoffrey Kaye with R.H.Orton and
D.G.Renton, 1946[60].

CKC 28: MARSHALL NITROUS
OXIDE-OXYGEN-ETHER
APPARATUS

Sir Geoffrey Marshall K.C.V.O. (Fig. 3.40), is now
the doyen of consulting physicians to Guy's
Hospital, London. In the First World War, he
served in the Royal Army Medical Corps on the
Western Front, and was particularly interested in
anaesthesia and the development of apparatus.
In 1917 he advocated the use of ether by Shipway's
apparatus (p. 185) for operations upon wounded
men[61].

While working with No. 17 Casualty Clearing
Station in France, from 1915 onwards, Marshall
made an apparatus for giving gas, oxygen and ether
with wet flowmeters. He was urged by Sir Anthony
Bowlby, the surgeon, to persuade an English manufacturer to produce a model. He got in touch with
Messrs Coxeter, who eventually produced a pro-
totype. This became a standard model in R.A.M.C.
practice. Marshall described it at a meeting of
the section of Anaesthetics at the Royal Society

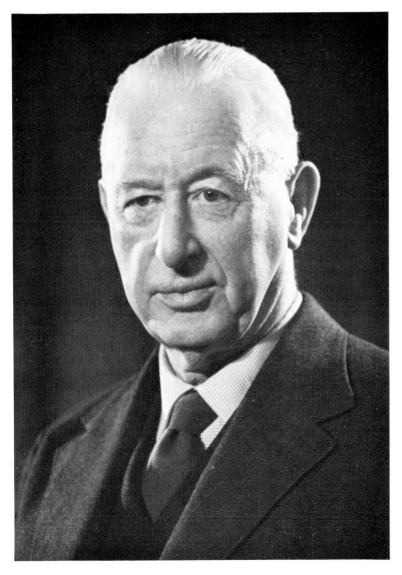

FIG. 3.40. SIR GEOFFREY MARSHALL
of Guy's Hospital.

of Medicine, though his papers show that early in 1917 he was advocating ether and chloroform by Shipway's apparatus (see p. 185), for abdominal injuries[63, 63]. The present apparatus was later discussed in Ross's textbook of 1919[64]. Before Marshall had published any account of the apparatus, Edmund Boyle of St Bartholomew's Hospital, then a Captain in the Royal Army Medical Corps, wrote the papers on his apparatus upon which he had worked for several years[65]. Thus the name of Boyle became for ever associated with this type of anaesthetic apparatus. The two 'heads' are almost identical, though both have the same construction as the earlier Gwathmey 'bubble-bottle' apparatus (see p. 142). The Marshall design consists of a plain bottle of about 300ml capacity with a rubber bung through which pass the two gas tubes (see Fig. 3.41). The bubble tubes are curved, to allow easy observation of the bubbles and each tube has six holes. The mixed gases are carried by a red rubber tube to the ether bottle, passing through a simple 'off-on' control which diverts them to the dip tube in the ether bottle. This dip tube has an elongating collar which may be adjusted to allow more bubbling to occur, though the extra depth in the specimen is of the order of $\frac{1}{4}''$ (0.6cm) only. A larger bore tube (though only of $\frac{7}{16}$ths of an inch, (1.1cm) diameter), carries the emitted gaseous mixture to the patient via a Hewitt stopcock with re-breathing bag. This is a relatively crudely made piece of apparatus, though fairly satisfactory in operation, in the context of its period. The improved design by Boyle, though little different, was undoubtedly slightly more sophisticated, especially in having reducing valves. Marshall's own paper did not come till 1920[66], when this apparatus was fully described by him at a meeting of the Section of Anaesthetics, Royal Society of Medicine. (Fig. 3.42). It was shown as a 'portable set' and a 'combined set', using identical heads.

FIG. 3.41 MARSHALL GAS-OXYGEN-ETHER APPARATUS, 1917. Head only. Curved tubes enter the bubble-bottle, which was borrowed from Gwathmey. The Coxeter ether control and larger bore delivery tube may be seen above the ether bottle.
CKC 28

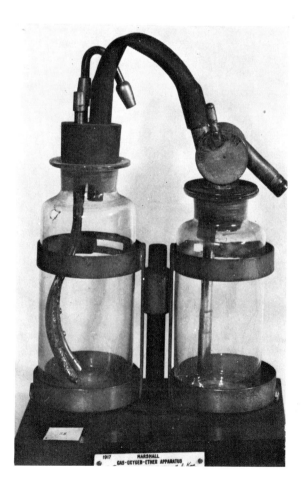

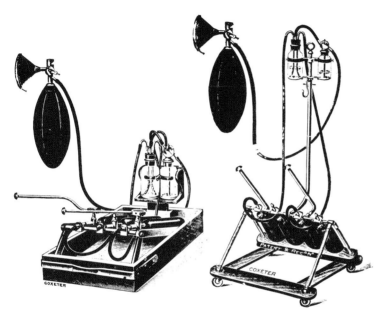

THE BOYLE APPARATUS

CKC 29   Boyle Nitrous Oxide/ oxygen/ether 1917

CKC 37   Boyle Nitrous Oxide/ oxygen/ether/chloroform 1926

CKC 39   Boyle nitrous oxide/ oxygen/ether/chloroform 1927

CKC 41   Boyle nitrous oxide/ oxygen/ether/chloroform 1930

CKC 44   Boyle nitrous oxide/ oxygen/ether/chloroform 1933

Henry Edmund Gaskin Boyle, 1875–1941 (Fig. 3.43), was born in Barbados, and qualified from St Bartholomew's Hospital, London in 1901[67]. He worked for a short time as Casualty Officer at Bristol Royal Infirmary, before returning to St Bartholomew's as Resident Anaesthetist. Boyle therefore received his early training in anaesthesia from Richard Gill, d. 1916, Foster Cross, 1873–1934, and others who had been brought up in the Clover era. The standard anaesthetic of the time consisted of a nitrous oxide induction using Cattlin's bag, followed by ether given from a Clover inhaler inserted between the bag and the face piece (see Fig. 1.25). These days and ways have been described by Hadfield in an interesting paper on Boyle[68]. As Hadfield says, Boyle and his contemporaries played an important part in bridging the gap between earlier methods and those which were to develop into the techniques of today; in surveying those years, it is now apparent that the great change began

FIG. 3.43. HENRY EDMUND
GASKIN BOYLE, 1875–1941,
of St Bartholomew's Hospital.

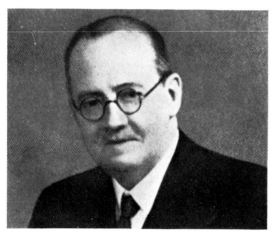

in the years immediately preceding the Great War and of course, during that War. We have already seen how Gwathmey (see p. 140) and Marshall (see p. 142) developed the use of nitrous oxide *with oxygen*, and produced a new method of gauging the gas flows. This was the idea which was then taken up by Boyle.

It was not Boyle's first attempt at the production of anaesthetic equipment. In 1912 he had described an apparatus for the intratracheal delivery of ether vapour, using a foot pump, a warm water bottle and an ether bottle (Fig. 3.44)[69]. It is thus easy to see that his mind was receptive to the idea which he saw Gwathmey use and which Marshall also copied. Boyle's original nitrous oxide/oxygen/ether apparatus of 1917, No. 29 in the Charles King Collection (Fig. 3.45) thus closely resembled those of Gwathmey and Marshall. The differences between this early Boyle and the Marshall (Fig. 3.41) are in detail only, and

the ether controls are similar, save only for the angles of the inflow and outflow tubes, which are more conveniently placed horizontally in Boyle's design. The control drums are identical and interchangeable, and the extension of the ether bubble tube is also present. Both were made by Messrs. Coxeter, who also designed the complete cylinder unit which was first fully described and figured by Boyle in the *Lancet*[70] and *British Medical Journal*[71] in 1919 (Figs. 3.46, 3.47). It was also presented to the Royal Society of Medicine in 1918. This appears to have been the first public appearance of the Boyle apparatus[72]. The features of this machine are the sight-feed and ether bottles, and the control (identical with the CKC 1917 specimen No. 29) mounted on a vertical rod: four nitrous oxide cylinders of 200 gallons each, with spirit lamp for warming the reducing valve: one oxygen cylinder of 20 cu. ft capacity: a small rebreathing bag and three-way stopcock with face piece. This is described as the hospital model, and variations were produced for use abroad and in private practice.

As the years passed, Boyle and the manufacturers, Messrs. Coxeter, modified and improved his apparatus. The model of 1926 (CKC 37, Fig. 3.48) differs from that of 1917 in its degree of sophistication. It has three bottles with bubble-tubes, five filler inlets with corks (of which two are air release ports), and a large-bore interconnecting mixing tube between the bottles, on the present day pattern.

The 1927 design (CKC 39, Fig. 3.49) has important developments. It is a three bottle version, the bottles again being connected in series by a mixing tube, and by a back-bar: a carbon dioxide sight feed tube has been added: the ether and chloroform bottles have lever controls, and the tubes in the bottles have two side holes and an end opening.

A similar model represents 1930 (CKC 41, Fig.

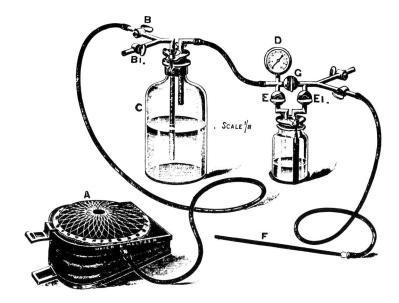

FIG. 3.44. BOYLE INTRATRACHEAL
INSUFFLATION APPARATUS, 1912,
for ether/air mixtures.
Described in Buxton,D.W. (1914)
Anaesthesia. London: Lewis, p. 197

3.50). Advances have been made by the provision of plungers in the chloroform and ether bottles, a significant improvement in control of vapour strength being thereby achieved: and by the addition of better fillers. The present example, No. 41, has a small-bore tube attached via a screw fitting to the outlet of the mixing tube. This appears to be a standard Boyle fitting of the period, being connected to a Cattlin reservoir bag (see Fig. 3.47). Though Magill had already made use of the widebore corrugated tube at this time, it does not seem to have been adopted by Boyle.

The model of 1933 (CKC 44, Fig. 3.51) made a significant advance with the adoption of Coxeter dry flow-meters, giving maximum flows of 18 litres nitrous oxide, 12 litres oxygen, and 6 litres carbon dioxide. The dry flow-meter consists of a bank of three tubes, each 20cm long and 8mm in diameter. These are mounted vertically close to each other inside a glass cylinder of 5cm diameter, in a protective metal case, sealed at each end by a metal collar and plate. No separate controls are provided, gas flows being adjusted by taps on the gas cylinder regulators. Each tube has twenty-four holes, and the rise of the dumb-bell shaped dry bobbin allows the gas to flow through those holes beneath it, into the larger glass cylinder. Variation in the maximum flows is achieved by making the twenty-four holes of larger diameter in the high flow nitrous oxide tube, smaller in the oxygen tube and smaller still in the

FIG. 3.45. BOYLE ORIGINAL GAS/
OXYGEN/ETHER HEAD, 1917.
Note the general similarity to the
Marshall apparatus (Fig. 3.41), and
to Gwathmey's (Fig. 3.39). It is
said that the first 'Boyle' was made
by Lord George Wellesley, while he
was an officer in the Royal Flying

Corps. Lord George became
managing director of Coxeters, and
a well-known designer of
anaesthetic equipment. He died in
1967 at the age of 78. (Obituary
notice. *Anaesthesia*, 1967, **22**, 710).
CKC 29

FIG. 3.46. BOYLE APPARATUS AS
SET UP.
The four cylinders have reducing
valves, and the mixture is piped
through the Cattlin bag. (Cf.
Marshall's apparatus, Fig. 3.41).
From *Lancet* 1919, **i**, 226

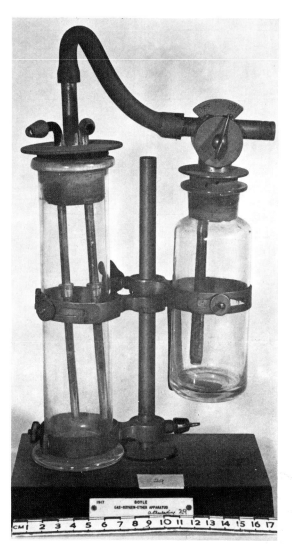

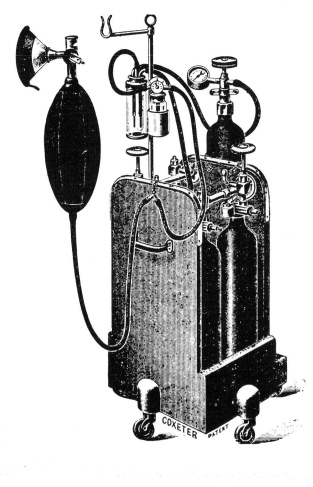

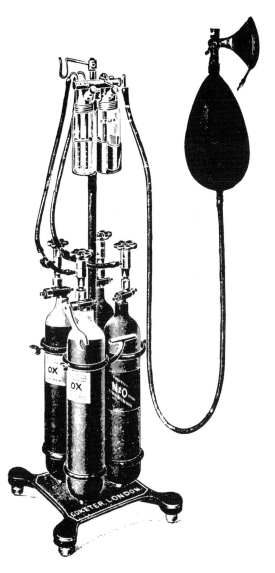

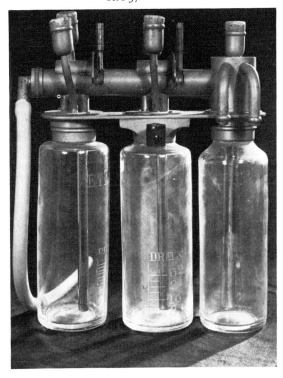

FIG. 3.48. BOYLE APPARATUS,
1926.
CKC 37

FIG. 3.47. BOYLE APPARATUS IN
ANOTHER VERSION.
Note the use of a Hewitt stopcock
between the face mask and the
Cattlin reservoir/rebreathing bag.
In this form, the apparatus was in
use throughout the 1930's.

FIG. 3.49. BOYLE APPARATUS,
1927.
Note the appearance of a carbon
dioxide 'bubble' tube, of lever
controls, and of a 'back-bar'.
CKC 39

FIG. 3.50. BOYLE APPARATUS,
1930.
'Plungers' have now been added.
CKC 41

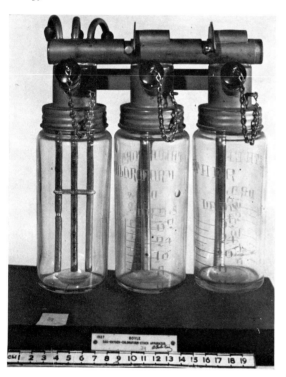

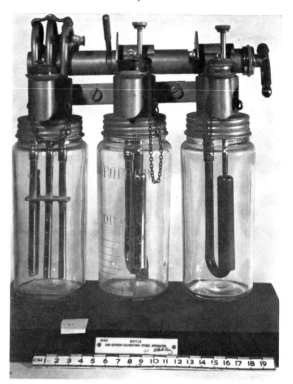

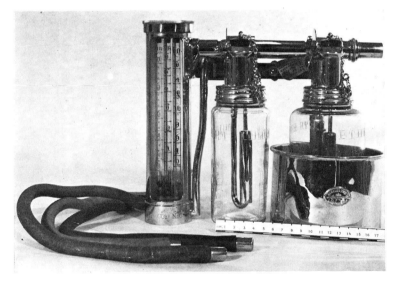

carbon dioxide tube.

The gases having mixed in the glass cylinder, pass through a hole in the base of the metal case into a vertical metal tube which carries them upwards to the large horizontal mixing tube, to which are attached the chloroform and ether bottles. These have control taps, and plungers which permit the escape of the mixed gases either above the level of the liquid or beneath its surface for higher concentrations of vapour. A water bath is usually provided for the ether bottle.

The dry-bobbin flowmeter of Messrs. Coxeter was an important step; reference will be made to the Siebe-Gorman flowmeters used by Magill in 1928 (see p. 195 and Fig. 4.19). Coxeter provided a practicable design incorporated in a head unit recognizable as the immediate forerunner of the modern anaesthetic apparatus. For this, H.E.G. Boyle had acted as the catalyst, obtaining the original idea from Gwathmey, seeing it used by Marshall and perhaps others, and pushing it forward by practical experiments and use.

Drs Alfred Lee and R. S. Atkinson give a useful resumé of the above development of the Boyle apparatus, which is so well demonstrated by the models in the Charles King Collection:

1917 Original Boyle, two gas water-sight feed (Fig. 3.45).

1920 Addition of vaporizing bottle to flowmeters.

1926 Addition of second vaporizing bottle and by-pass controls. (Fig. 3.48).

1927 Addition of third water-sight feed tube for carbon dioxide. (Fig. 3.49).

1930 Addition of plunger device. (Fig. 3.50).

1933 Dry-bobbin type of flow-meter displaced water sight-feed. (Fig. 3.51).

1937 Rotameters displaced dry-bobbin flow-meters[73].

FIG. 3.52. SHIPWAY APPARATUS, 1920.
Head only.
CKC 30

CKC 30: SHIPWAY NITROUS OXIDE, OXYGEN, ETHER APPARATUS 1920

Evidence of the interest in the developments produced by Gwathmey and Boyle is shown by those who copied their designs, usually with minor alterations only. Among these are the next two pieces to be described.

That of Shipway (CKC 30, Fig. 3.52) was produced in 1920. Shipway, anaesthetist to Guy's Hospital, had already brought out his warm ether 'blow-over' apparatus and it is by this that he is best remembered. This is described on a later page (see p. 185).* The present piece is lesser known and is a curious mixture of Shipway's earlier apparatus and of a modified Boyle head.

Nitrous oxide and oxygen are passed through the usual water-sight feed bottle after the manner of Gwathmey and Boyle. The mixture passes to an unusual ether bottle, set in a water bath; the control tap (Fig. 3.53) allows direct passage of the gases, or in an intermediate position, deflects a small amount into the ether bottle. Placing the tap in the E (ether) position however, cuts off the gas-flow, and air ether vapour is then drawn over by the patient through one of two other tubes in the bottle cap. The smaller of these, D, has a tap fitted to it; the larger, C, seems not to have had anything connected to it and so is open to the air. These tubes are short, only reaching below the cap of the ether bottle: the main gas tube passes to the bottom and is open at its lower end, with a group of eight small holes immediately above.

The functions of the two shorter tubes, C and D, are not readily explicable, though it is possible that the larger was the air-inlet of a draw-over system,

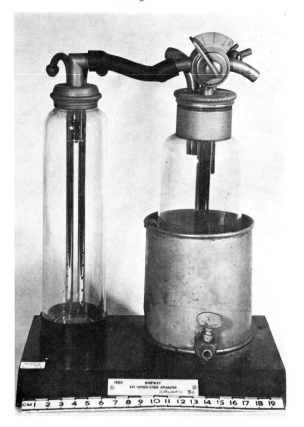

Shipway being given to this type of apparatus (see Nos. 25. 26. p. 185). It is unusual in that turning the control tap to the full ether position, closes the gas/oxygen inlet A. The smaller tube D was perhaps intended for an extra oxygen supply.

The apparatus in complete form was described by Shipway to the Section of Anaesthetics of the Royal Society of Medicine in 1920[74]. The head is shown clamped to a rod on a cylinder stand. The ether

* The two are described as *similar* in my inventory, *Anaesthesia*. 1970. **25**. 557. This is not correct. K.B.T.

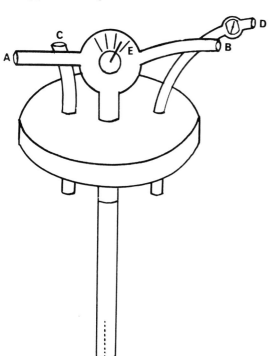

FIG. 3.53. CONTROL, SHIPWAY
GAS, OXYGEN, ETHER APPARATUS,
1920
A. Inlet for gases.
B. To patient.
C. ? Draw-over tube.
D. ? Extra oxygen inlet.
E. Ether control tap—in the 'off'
   position only the gases flow. In
   intermediate position $N_2O/O_2/$
   ether is delivered. In E position,
   the gases are cut off, and ether
   only passes to the patient via B.

bottle is simpler than that on the King Collection example, lacking the tubes C and D. Delivery to the face mask is via a narrow-bore tube and Hewitt's stopcock with Cattlin type rebreathing bag, (Fig. 3.54), but the gases pass directly to the face piece, and not into the bag, an innovation and improvement which Marshall had also used (see Fig. 3.42).

CKC 31: WEBBER NITROUS OXIDE-OXYGEN-ETHER-CHLOROFORM APPARATUS 1920

Harald Norris Webber, 1881–1954[75] worked at University College Hospital, London. With his colleague Felix Stephens Rood, 1883–1933, he wrote an unconventional and somewhat trite textbook in 1930[76], from which a quotation regarding the use of adrenaline with chloroform, is given elsewhere (see p. 64).

Webber worked with the psychologist W.H.R. Rivers, at Cambridge, whose Croonian lecture on alcohol was published in 1908. As Webber was a confirmed teetotaler, he had been an ideal subject, and the lecture was based on experiments made on him! In 1948 he was elected as one of the first Fellows of the newly established Faculty of Anaesthetists. His obituary notice states that his apparatus of 1920 was then (1955) still in use at University College Hospital.

Webber's apparatus (Fig. 3.55) consists of three bottles grouped below the mixing chamber into which run the gas tubes. The ether and chloroform bottles are set in parallel instead of in series, as in Boyle and Marshall's apparatus, thus preventing the carrying over of chloroform vapour into the ether bottle. The mixing chamber is prolonged into a double tube on the forward end of which is the dial

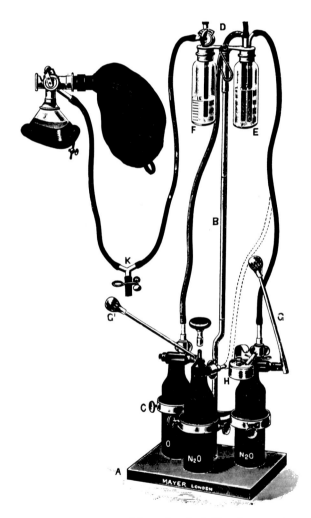

FIG. 3.54. SHIPWAY APPARATUS
AS SET UP.
From *Proc. Roy. Soc. Med.* (1920)
13, Pt I (*Anaesth Section*) p. 20

A, wooden base; **B**, upright rod; **C**, holder for cylinders; **D**, unit;
E, mixing chamber; **F**, ether bottle; **G, G**, levers; **H**, spirit lamp; **K**, water-
trap.

FIG. 3.55. WEBBER THREE-BOTTLE
DELIVERY HEAD, 1920.
Oxygen, carbon dioxide and nitrous
oxide connecting tubes at back.
Below the rotating control is the
small-bore delivery tube.
CKC 31

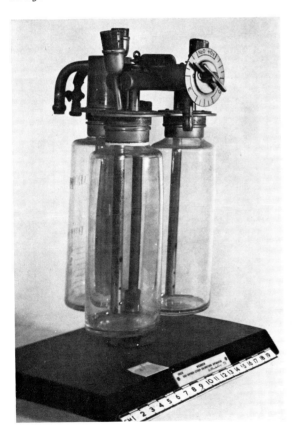

control; this rotates the inner tube which has ports reminiscent of those of a Clover apparatus (Fig. 3.56), allowing any combination of vapours to be delivered. The chloroform and ether bottles, right and left in front, have dip-tubes with two small holes at their lower ends and a larger hole above. Three gas inlets allow for nitrous oxide, oxygen and carbon dioxide, and the water-sight feed tubes are complex, that for CO_2 being straight with five side holes, that for nitrous oxide being returned on itself as a U, to provide in all eleven holes, while the oxygen tube, with five lower holes, has also a side-tube at the upper end, to which a piece of glass tubing has been attached. These complicated tortuosities merely provide more scope for the volume of gases passed through. The mixture outlet is of narrow bore and the gases were probably passed to a Cattlin reservoir bag before reaching the face mask.

CKC 32: McKESSON NITROUS OXIDE/OXYGEN APPARATUS, MODEL G, 1920
CKC 60: NARGRAF MODEL J, c 1930

Elmer Isaac McKesson, 1881–1935, (Fig. 3.57) of Toledo, Ohio, was a distinguished American anaesthetist, who had considerable influence on anaesthesia in the United States between the two World wars. He was a leading figure, with Francis McMechan, in the formation of the Interstate Association of Anaesthetists[77], but he was better known in this country for two innovations, one aberrant, and one of practical use, the McKesson apparatus.

McKesson was undoubtedly aberrant in the introduction of his 'secondary saturation' technique, though it produced more than a passing interest, and a good deal of controversy. Gwathmey[78] used

FIG. 3.56. CONTROL TUBE OF
WEBBER NITROUS OXIDE/
OXYGEN/CHLOROFORM/ETHER
APPARATUS.
The tube has been pulled out from
the head to show the ports which

engage corresponding holes in the
outer tube. The small-bore delivery
tube lies below the control tube.
The use of the latter enables the
bottles to be set up in parallel.

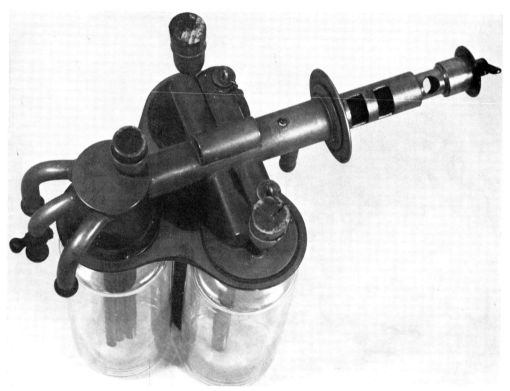

a heading 'DOUBLE SATURATION CON-
DEMNED', and considered it to be 'an unphysio-
logical and dangerous process.' McKesson's account
plainly confirmed this assertion, though he himself
would not have it so. After description of the initial
saturation with 100 per cent nitrous oxide, with subsequent addition of a little oxygen, McKesson
described 'Secondary saturation. Reduce the proportion of oxygen or administer 100 per cent nitrous
oxide until the pupil dilates and tonic muscular
spasm or rigidity develops, and respiration becomes

slow or stops. Now administer one breath of 75 to
100 per cent oxygen, if he inhales; if he does not,
partly fill the lungs by inflation with pure oxygen
once or twice. . . . The cyanotic colour now begins
to lighten, the pupils retract, the pulse is normal or
slower than before, the muscles become perfectly relaxed and presently respirations resume.' McKesson
added 'I believe this is safer for a patient than an
ether sequence or combined gas oxygen-ether mixture, and convalescence is decidedly better when
even the small amount of combined ether is

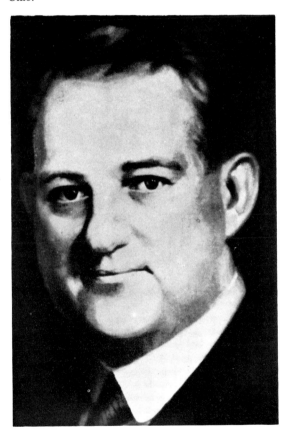

McKesson's low oxygen percentage technique.

In a later paper[81], read to the Section of Anaesthetics at the Royal Society of Medicine in 1926, McKesson somewhat modified his position, largely, as he admitted, because his first paper had described the 'rapid method' which 'had done nothing but scare people': so he described the 'slow method' which consisted in 'merely cutting down the oxygen percentage by perhaps one or two per cent, and continuing the narcosis until the accumulation of nitrous oxide produces signs of anoxaemia.' However, at this same meeting, H.E.G.Boyle said that he had seen Dr McKesson perform secondary saturation, and candidly it had scared him.

On the other hand McKesson's nitrous oxide apparatus was enthusiastically received. The original model was described in 1911[82] and its development over the next twenty years or so has almost an epic quality. The paper of 1911 described a nitrous oxide/oxygen sequence, with insistence upon carbon dioxide rebreathing as a safe and desirable procedure. McKesson quoted the papers of Yandell Henderson, the American pioneer of respiratory physiology, whose views on the control of respiration by carbon dioxide were given in a later paper to the Dental Board of the United Kingdom[83]. Yandell Henderson advocated the use of 'a controllable amount of rebreathing', and McKesson therefore designed his first apparatus to retain a portion of each exhalation in the rebreathing bag, the remainder escaping into the atmosphere. He wrote 'As much fresh gas is inhaled at the next breath as escaped before, so a constant controllable amount of rebreathing is possible. . . .'[82], and 'fractional rebreathing', as he named it, was one of the mainstays of his anaesthetic designs.

This however, was not McKesson's major con-

avoided. . . .'[79] These views were of course, sincerely held, and the writer remembers as a young house anaesthetist, tales told by his seniors of demonstrations by McKesson in London, when completely cyanotic patients became pink and relaxed on flooding with oxygen. The technique was not, to his knowledge, in use at that time (*c.* 1939), but no violent condemnation is recalled, and Stanley Sykes[80] in 1935 actually defended tribution to the development of apparatus, for he was also the initiator of the method of intermittent flow. In 1926, in a valuable paper to the Section of Anaesthetics at the British Medical Association Annual Meeting at Nottingham[84], he discussed the function and design of anaesthetic apparatus based on the principles of respiratory physiology, as then envisaged. Here he gave four main functions for an anaesthetic apparatus; firstly, the design of proper components; secondly, proper control of the mixture of gases; thirdly, control of the pressure of the mixed gases; fourthly, the regulation of re-breathing. His third function of pressure control was to give rise to the intermittent flow principle. He was somewhat critical of the 'water type gas meter' as described by Gwathmey and others, which pro-vided a continuous flow. McKesson wrote under the heading *The Intermittent Flow Method*: 'After con-siderable clinical experience with various forms of mixing apparatus then available, I experimented along another line. The mechanical problem presented many difficulties, but it appeared that if the nitrous oxide and oxygen bags could be kept equally filled or under equal but very low pressure by some automatic bag filling mechanism, progress might be made. After several trials, such valves were perfected which automatically replenished the oxygen and the nitrous oxide bags at each breath, stopping the flow from the tanks into the bags while the patient exhaled and paused between breaths. The bags were thus kept equally filled . . . regard-less of the rate or volume of respirations . . . the two bags were placed together in a bag of fish net so that any, even very slight, differences of pressure of the two gases within the bags would be equalised by their walls pressing against each other. The pressure in the two bags was then always equal. . . . Instead of a continuous flow apparatus this became an intermittent flow device. Certain advantages resulted, among which were a foundation for proper mixture control and relief from attempts at manually adjust-ing the rate of flow, since the respirations regulated this function much better than the anaesthetist had done before. The possible range of gas delivery was enormous—from nothing to more than 33 gallons a minute, so that no patient could exhaust the supply, however rapidly he breathed. The intermittent flow principle also adapted itself to the technique for intermittent administration in producing analgesia for obstetrics'[84].

Both McKesson machines in the Charles King Collection are of this type, the earlier (No. 32) being dated by King to 1920: the later (No. 60) presented to the Collection in 1966 by the late Dr Ronald Jarman, is of more advanced design, and is described in detail in a booklet published by Charles King in 1930[85] (Fig. 3.58).

The 1920 apparatus, model G, (Figs. 3.59, 3.60, 3.61) has four cylinder yokes with two reducing valves registering 120 lbs/sq in. Reinforced rubber tubing leads from each valve to a mixing chamber with a mixture control dial calibrated for nitrous oxide/air or nitrous oxide/oxygen in any proportions. On the front of the mixing chamber is mounted an ether vaporizer with gutta-percha heat insulation, (Fig. 3.59) and a wide-bore tube leads to the face piece with expiratory valve (missing from the specimen).

Twin reservoir bags are mounted side by side beneath the main casting, in a single fishnet bag. McKesson had written of the equalizing of pressure established by this arrangement, but one may doubt how far this was really so. He himself, on the same page had remarked that 'Hewett's (sic) two bags having a common rubber partition was probably not an attempt to equalise pressures, as there is no such

FIG. 3.58. TITLE PAGE OF
BOOKLET
published in 1930 by Charles King.

McKesson Nargraf

for

General Anæsthesia

Copyright 1930—McKesson Appliance Company, Toledo, Ohio, U.S.A.

*Please add this to your file
of Anæsthetic Papers.*

*Should you not have copies
of our recent Addenda please
apply for them.*

A. CHARLES KING, Ltd.
34, Devonshire Street
Harley Street
London, W.1

Telephone : Welbeck 2264 (2 lines).
Telegrams : Analgesia, Wesdo, London.
Cablegrams : Analgesia, London.

FIG. 3.59. MCKESSON, MODEL G,
1920.
Note metal clamps beside gas-bag,
with tension spring, and ether
vaporizer with insulation. (Cf. Fig.
3.60). Each reducing valve has two
cylinder attachments.
CKC 32

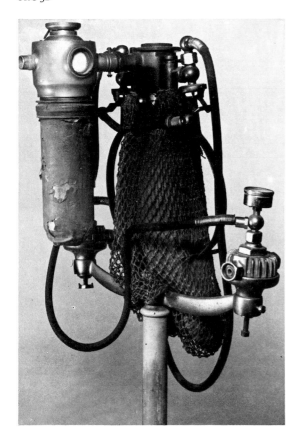

purpose found in the literature, and they certainly
could not have so functioned.' It is notable that the
idea was dropped from later McKesson models.

A movable curved metal bar, or clamp, extends
down the side of each bag (Figs. 3.59, 3.60) being connected to a check valve which reduces the gas intake
as the bag expands to move the clamp. The two
clamps are themselves connected by a spring and
screw which tightens the bags against each other,
and so controls the pressure within each bag. By
combining this manoeuvre with opening or closing
the expiratory valve, it was possible to control the
degree of rebreathing, to provide 'fractional rebreathing', and to obtain intermittent flow.

The McKesson Nargraf, Model J, for nitrous
oxide/oxygen, first appeared about 1930, and has
remained in use for many years. It is a refined version
of the Model G described above. (Figs. 3.62, 3.63,
3.64). The mixing chamber now has a glass topped
control providing 0–100 per cent oxygen with nitrous
oxide, and a direct oxygen button is added. The gas
bags are protected in metal cases, and a pressure
control allows pressures of 0–40mmHg, by adjust-
ing the tension on a check valve mounted in the
main casting; this in turn is connected by a central
rod and two pivoted arms to the gas-bags in their
metal cases (Fig. 3.64). Fractional rebreathing
is obtained via an oblong concertina bag at the rear
of the mount. A clock key rotates a dial on the side
indicating a pressure of 0–12mmHg. King's leaflet
states 'in practice this is made to equal the pressure
of the gases administered to the patient'; in the
limited experience of the present author using this
apparatus, this was not easy to achieve. The machines
also varied greatly from one to another. A stop for
the rebreathing bag is provided, with an indicator
dial showing the volume of the rebreathed gases.

The McKesson apparatus represented a real

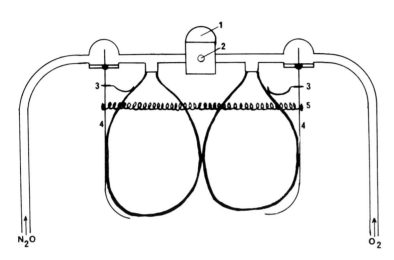

FIG. 3.60. SKETCH OF MODEL G
MCKESSON.
1. Mixing chamber and control.
2. To patient.
3. Check valves.
4. Clamps acting on check-valves.
5. Tension spring between clamps
   increases pressure equally in the
   gas bags.

advance in physiological and precision anaesthesia,
and it achieved wide acceptance and popularity;
Mennell described it as 'the Rolls Royce of nitrous
oxide machines'[86]. It was set up in various forms
and King's Catalogue shows the cost of the hospital
model (Fig. 3.65) as £126. 4. 0; a high price in the
day of the voluntary hospital, when anaesthesia
could be produced with a rag and a bottle of ether.

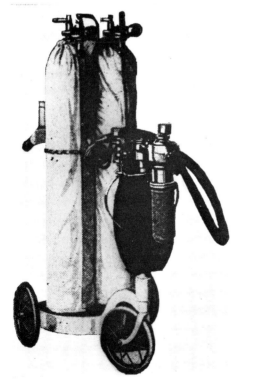

FIG. 3.61. MCKESSON MODEL G.
as mounted for hospital use.
From Gwathmey, J.T. (1914)
Anesthesia. New York: Appleton,
p. 151

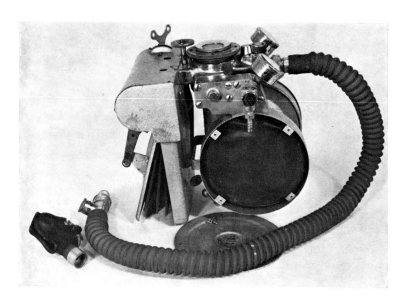

FIG. 3.62. McKESSON MODEL J,
1930, WITH NARGRAF HEAD.
Behind the corrugated tube outlet is
the knurled pressure control, and
behind this, the large oxygen
percentage dial, with a fine control
also. One panel has been removed
to show the rubber nitrous oxide
demand regulator bag, on the inner
side of which is a pivoted arm
connected to the central check valve.
(Cf. Figs. 3.67 and 3.68). At the
rear is the concertina rebreathing
bag, the pressure in which may be
controlled by the key.
CKC 60

CKC 72: WALTON I NITROUS OXIDE/ OXYGEN MACHINE 1925

with

CKC 56: Self administering analgesia

and

CKC 57: Ethyl chloride attachments for Walton II (1938)

The Walton I machine (Fig. 3.66) for dental nitrous oxide/oxygen was the first British intermittent flow apparatus. Apocryphally, the name is said to have been conjured up during a game of golf at a well-known course, and the apparatus continued in this form until the advent of the Walton II in 1938, though it is probably still giving useful, if outmoded, service in some dental surgeries.

The essential of the Walton intermittent demand control is quite simple and may be compared with that of the McKesson machine. The gases pass to separate bags from the cylinders. As the bags inflate, they cause a cranked pinchcock to occlude the supply tube. Inhalation reduces the bag pressure and gas thereupon flows into it. Fig. 3.67 shows the principle with a concertina bag as applied to the Walton II. The Walton I used balloon bags of 2 litre capacity. From the bags the gases passed to a mixing stopcock, which could be set to deliver any percentage mixture of nitrous oxide/oxygen or nitrous oxide/air (Fig. 3.68). The gas control was by foot pedal moving from low pressure to high pressure, again by pinching the supply tube. Nitrous oxide/oxygen percentages were stated by the manufacturers, British Oxygen Company, to be accurate at all pressures, though nitrous oxide/air mixtures were only accurate when the gas was

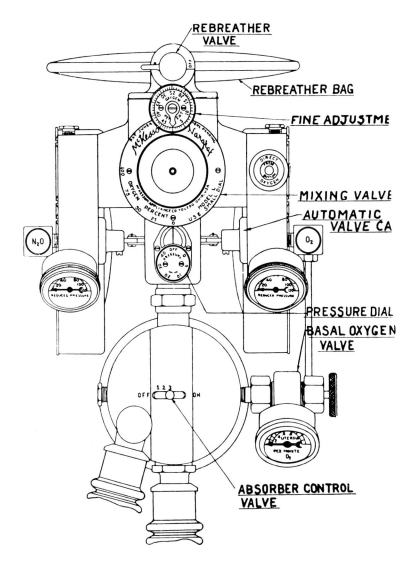

REBREATHER
VALVE

REBREATHER BAG

FINE ADJUSTME

MIXING VALVE

AUTOMATIC
VALVE CA

PRESSURE DIAL

BASAL OXYGEN
VALVE

ABSORBER CONTROL
VALVE

N₂O

O₂

FIG. 3.63. DIAGRAM OF MCKESSON
MODEL J. FROM ABOVE.
From Charles King's pamphlet,
1930.

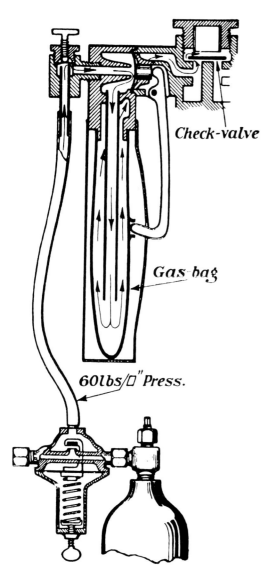

FIG. 3.64. DIAGRAM OF MCKESSON
MODEL J,
showing gas-bag, check valve, and
lever, the principle of the
demand regulator.
From Charles King's Pamphlet,
1930.

Check-valve

Gas-bag

60lbs/□" Press.

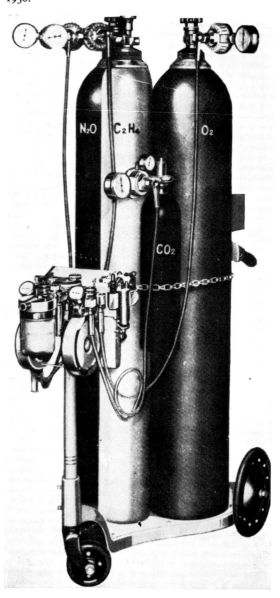

FIG. 3.65. MCKESSON MODEL J. AS
SET UP FOR HOSPITAL USE.
The apparatus as here arranged
somewhat resembled in
manœuvreability a three-wheeled
tramcar. An example remained in
use, to the author's knowledge, until
the 1960's.
From Charles King's pamphlet,
1930.

FIG. 3.66. WALTON I. NITROUS
OXIDE/OXYGEN APPARATUS, 1925.
The foot pedal, operating through a
rod, controls the gas flows to the
mixing chamber, where the oxygen
percentage may be adjusted. As the
bags fill, the gas flows are
interrupted by pinchcocks attached
to the curved levers. The mixture
passes via a lever control, either to
the corrugated tube, or to the
double tubes and a Goldman nose
piece.
CKC 72

FIG. 3.67. PRINCIPLE OF THE
WALTON INTERMITTENT FLOW
APPARATUS.

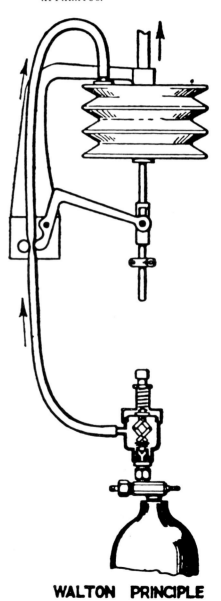

WALTON PRINCIPLE

delivered at low pressure. In 1967, Nainby-Luxmoore[87] pointed out that the accuracy of intermittent flow machines is greatly dependent on frequent servicing, and latterly there has been a move away from these to continuous flow machines in dental and out-patient departments.

Various additions and attachments were designed for the Walton machines, of which Models III (1946), IV (1955), V (1958) were subsequent designs. Thus ether bottles, trichlorethylene and halothane vaporizers have been added, and an oro-nasal inhaler was produced for use with the Walton II though a double oral/oro-nasal unit was much used with the Walton I (Fig. 3.68).

The King Collection has an ethyl chloride attachment (No. 57, Fig. 3.69). A graduated test tube allowed ethyl chloride to be run into a special bag inserted between the corrugated tube and the face mask; a non-return valve was fitted to prevent contamination of the corrugated tube by ethyl chloride.

A further attachment (No. 56, Fig. 3.70) is the self-administering analgesia attachment, for use in the dental surgery. This was plugged in to the mixing stopcock. The Walton was then set to deliver a predetermined mixture of nitrous oxide/air. The control on top of the attachment has three settings. At 'full control', the pre-set mixture is delivered so long as the patient keeps a rubber bulb compressed. Upon release of this pressure, only air is delivered. At 'gas limited', gas diluted with air is administered, but release of the bulb delivers air only. At the 'air limited' setting, the pre-set mixture

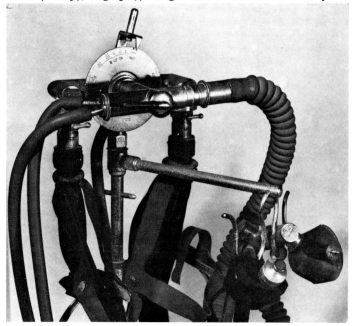

FIG. 3.68. WALTON I STOPCOCK SHOWING PERCENTAGE SETTINGS.
The same stopcock continued in use for later models. Both delivery tubes have nose pieces fitted. The rubber straps prevent over distension of the bags, but the latter are not now inflatable.
CKC 72

FIG. 3.69. ETHYL CHLORIDE
ATTACHMENT
originally designed for use with
Walton II (1938).
CKC 57

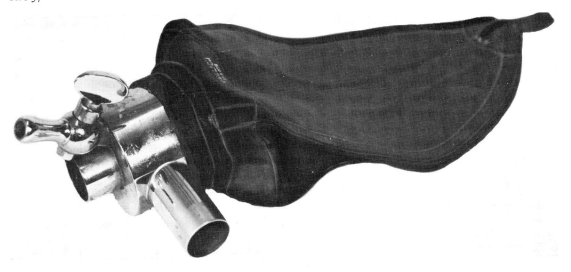

FIG. 3.70. SELF-ADMINISTERING
ANALGESIA ATTACHMENT
for Walton II. (1938).
A hand bellows was attached to
the tube at lower end. The patient
compressed the bellows until
supervening unconsciousness
caused release when air alone
entered.
CKC 56

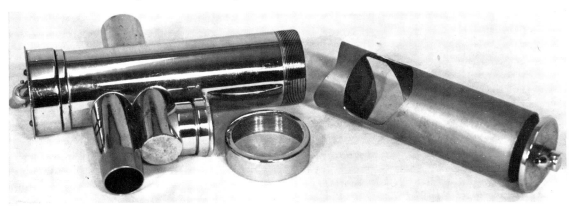

is inhaled, till release of the bulb allows a dilute nitrous oxide/air mixture to be given. The manufacturers pamphlet states 'with experience, this attachment used in conjunction with the Walton mixture control, is an extremely comprehensive apparatus, with which the anaesthetist can obtain any degree of analgesia or anaesthesia'[88].

Anaesthetists who made use of this apparatus were possibly not quite so sanguine as to such delicacy and ease of control, and the Walton analgesia system did not acquire the popularity of the Minnitt gas/air machine.

CKC 71: CONNELL NITROUS OXIDE/ OXYGEN ABSORBER APPARATUS 1937

Karl Connell (d. 1941), was Instructor in Surgery, Columbia University, at the time when he described an ether vaporizer with a measured air stream carrying over the ether vapour[89]. The vaporizer was warmed on an electric stove! Among other anaesthetic apparatus were his double nasopharyngeal tubes[90], and in an obituary note his death is described as causing a genuine loss in the entire field of anaesthesiology[91].

The present apparatus was given to the Collection by Dr Massey Dawkins, University College Hospital, who had it in use from 1937 until a very recent date. The apparatus is housed in an elegant stainless steel wheeled cabinet—an early date for the use of this material. Three drawers and an open space occupy the lower part and the top shelf carries the apparatus itself.

A typed pamphlet accompanies the machine (Fig. 3.71), containing also a diagram of the circuits (Fig. 3.72). An important feature of the apparatus is the well-known Connell ballbearing flowmeter,

FIG. 3.71. CONNELL APPARATUS, 1937.
CKC 71

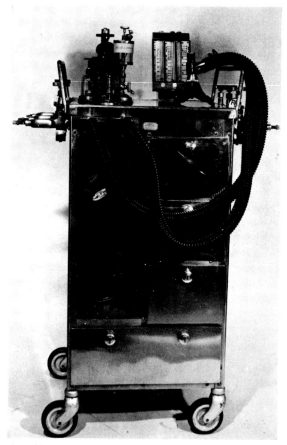

described thus:

'Flow Meters, U.S. Patent, July 3, 1934
The meter tube is of K.P. Jena glass of tapered interior formed on Zeiss precision mandrels and accurate to the ten thousandth of an inch. The taper is compound so that all useful readings, both fine and course, are condensed in a short space. The fine taper increases a thousandth of an inch in diameter for

every inch in length, giving readings over the first three inches of excursion accurate to 10 c.c. of gas per minute.'

The upper taper is parabolic and is increasingly fast, giving readings on larger flow volumes such as are useful for induction and for straight flow methods and emergency flow.

The moving member of the flowmeter is the tandem of two stainless steel balls, very sensitive and of size accurate to one ten-thousandth of an inch. (*The diameter is 4mm.* K.B.T.). The reading is taken from the line of contact between the two balls.

All parts of the meter are visible and readily cleaned. The balls seat below on a stainless steel coil spring and are limited in upper excursion by a recoil bumper so that large and emergency volumes may be rushed through without recourse to treacherous by-passes' (Fig. 3.73).

The pamphlet also contains the following interesting passage:

'*History of Connell Flow Meters*
The Connell apparatus of 1908 was the first apparatus to carry precise measurement of anaesthetic gases. The kinetic flow meters employed in this apparatus were of the piston type. In the model of 1912 and the War model of 1917 these pistons were superceded by a rotary vane type of flow gauge, a delicate vane mounted on gold pinions in jewel bearings. In 1925 Dr Connell again became interested to devise a shock-proof meter of exceeding accuracy. The present superior flow meter entered the Connell Model A of 1930, a custom built apparatus of the fractional rebreathing type and of advanced design. The ball flow meter as now constructed is the most sensitive, accurate and compact dry flow-meter as yet devised. It is a method practically trouble proof and everlasting. Fine flows, coarse flows, and emergency volumes of gas may be passed through the same meter without damage to its sensitiveness. By-passes,

necessary in other apparatus, are treacherous and prone to leak and have no place in the Connell machine.'

The priority claimed for the precise measurement of gases in 1908 is probably true so far as anaesthetic apparatus is concerned. The experimental bubble-bottle of Cotton and Boothby (1912), was adopted by Gwathmey in the same year (see p. 141). Details of Connell's 'Kinetic flow meter' of 1908 do not seem to be available.

The flowmeter panel on the present model (Fig. 3.73) has three inclined tubes, each with a pair of ballbearings, from the junction of which the reading is taken. One tube registers oxygen, being calibrated from 50 cc/min to 8 litres, the second shows two gas markings, carbon dioxide to 500 cc/min with helium, 1 to 10 litres, in its upper segment; the third tube is marked 'for anaesthetic gases'. The calibrating panel for this tube may be rotated: one side shows markings for cyclopropane and nitrous oxide, 50 cc–8 litres/min, the same calibrations being used; the other side is marked for ethylene, 50 cc–8 litres/min, with a separate set of red calibrations for helium, 100 cc–10 litres/min.

Such a multiplicity of gases must at least have made confusion possible, particularly as the cylinder yokes, as was usual in those days, were not 'keyed', and cylinders were thus interchangeable.

There are no reducing valves, but fine adjustment valves are arranged above the cylinder yokes. The remainder of the apparatus is set neatly upon the upper table and consists of light-weight non-return valves set under two glass domes, soda lime cannister marked with 'hours of use' and a drip-bottle, nominally for ether, but now marked 'fluothane'. There is an adjustable safety-valve and two corrugated patient tubes with a two-litre reservoir bag. All the internal gas connections are

permanently fitted with soldered copper tubing, and
the whole apparatus is a fine piece of anaesthetic
engineering.

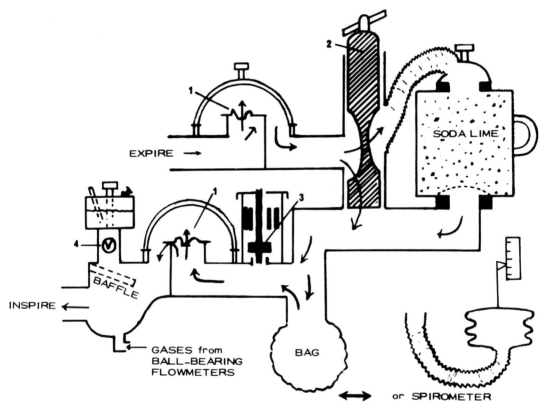

FIG. 3.72. SCHEME OF CONNELL
APPARATUS, 1937.
From a diagram in the descriptive
pamphlet.
1 Unidirectional flutter valves,
   beneath glass domes. The 'flutter
   unit' is a corrugated rubber disc,
   vulcanized to a central disc of
silver and mounted on a stainless
steel bearing.
2 Soda lime shunt valve.
3 Weighted spill valve.
4 Ether dropper.

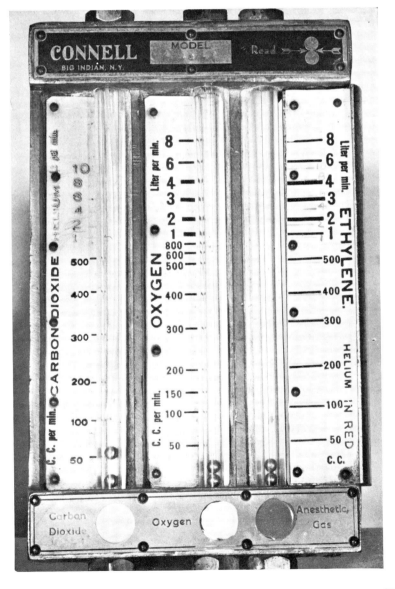

FIG. 3.73. BALL-BEARING
FLOWMETERS
of Connell apparatus, 1937.
The tubes are 16cm in length and
have a compound taper. The panel
for anaesthetic gases shows the
calibrations for helium and ethylene.
It may be rotated to show those for
nitrous oxide and cyclopropane.

REFERENCES

1 SMITH W.D.A. (1965). (1972) A History of Nitrous Oxide and Oxygen Anaesthesia. Pt. I. *Brit. J. Anaesth.* **37**. 790. Pt. IA. *Brit. J. Anaesth.* **44**. 297.

2 PRIESTLEY J. (1776) *Experiments and observations on different kinds of air.* London: Johnson. 2nd ed. p. 45.

3 BARZUN J. (1972) Thomas Beddoes or Medicine and Social Conscience. *J. Amer. med. Ass.* **220**. 51.

4 [BEDDOES T.] (1790) *Chemical Experiments and Opinions extracted from a work published in the last century.*

5 GOODWYN E. (1788). *The Connection of Life with Respiration: or an experimental inquiry into the effects of submersion, strangulation and several kinds of noxious airs on animals.* London: Johnson.

6 BEDDOES T, (1793) *Letter to Erasmus Darwin, M.D., on a new method of treating pulmonary consumption.* Bristol: Bulgin and Rosser.

7 CARTWRIGHT F.F. (1951) *The English Pioneers of Anaesthesia.* Bristol: Wright.

8 BEDDOES T. (1797) *Reports principally concerning the Effects of the Nitrous Acid in the Venereal Disease, by the Surgeons of The Royal Hospital at Plymouth.* London: Johnson.

9 BEDDOES T. and WATT J. (1794–96) *Considerations on the Medicinal Use and the Production of Factitious Airs.* London: Johnson.

10 BEDDOES T. (1799) *Notice of some Observations made at the Medical Pneumatic Institution.* Bristol: Biggs and Cottle.

11 DAVY H. (1800) *Researches, Chemical and Philosophical, chiefly concerning Nitrous Oxide or Dephlogisticated Nitrous Air and its Respiration.* London: Johnson. p. 453 (facsimile reproduction. London: Butterworths. 1972).

12 DAVY H. (1800) *ibid.* p. 465, p. 556.

13 DAVY H. (1800) *ibid.* p. 471.

14 BARTON W.P.C. (1808) *Dissertation on the Chemical Properties and exhilarating effects of nitrous gas: and its application to pneumatic medicine.* Thesis for the degree of Doctor of Medicine. Philadelphia.

15 [FARADAY M.] (1818) On the effects of inhaling the vapour of sulphuric ether. *J. Science and Arts.* Royal Institution. London. **4**. 158.

16 SMITH W.D.A. (1965) A History of Nitrous Oxide and Oxygen Anaesthesia, Pt. II. *Brit. J. Anaesth.* **37**. 879.

17 DUNCUM B. (1947) *The Development of Inhalation Anaesthesia.* London: Oxford Univ. Press. p. 94.

18 KIDD C. (1864) The New Anaesthetic—nitrous oxide. *Med. Times & Gaz.* **i**. 301.

19 DUNCUM B. (1947) *op. cit.* p. 285 et seq.

20 SMITH W.D.A. (1966) A History of Nitrous Oxide and Oxygen Anaesthesia. Pt. VII. 1868— Nitrous Oxide takes root in Great Britain. *Brit. J. Anaesth.* **38**. 551.

21 SMITH W.D.A. (1966) A History of Nitrous Oxide and Oxygen. Pt. IX. *Brit. J. Anaesth.* **38**. 950.

22 COTTON F.J. and BOOTHBY W.M. (1912) Nitrous oxide-oxygen-ether anaesthesia. *Surgery, Gynaecology, Obstetrics.* **15**. 281–289.

23 GWATHMEY J.T. (1925) *Anesthesia.* Macmillan: New York. 2nd ed. p. 153.

24 JACKSON D.E. (1915) New Method for the Production of General Analgesia and Anaesthesia. *J. Laboratory and Clinical Medicine.* **1**. 1–12.

25 CRILE G. and LOWER W.E. (1914) *Anoci-Association.* Saunders. Philadelphia.

26 PARBROOK G.D. (1970) Nitrous Oxide Toxicity, in *Progress in Anaesthesiology,* ed. Boulton et al. Excerpta Medica. Amsterdam. p. 316.

27 RYMER S.L. (1864) Remarks upon the Use of Nitrous Oxide in Dental operations. *Dental Review.* N.S. I. 1–9.

28 SMITH W.D.A. (1970) The Development of Nitrous Oxide Anaesthesia. In *Progress in Anaesthesiology.* Proceedings of the 4th World Congress of Anaesthesiologists. 1968. ed. Boulton et al. Amsterdam. p. 209.

29 *A Century of Service to Dentistry, 1844–1944.* (1944).

S.S.White Dental Mfg. Co. Philadelphia.

30 CLOVER J.T. (1876) An Apparatus for Administering Nitrous Oxide Gas and Ether, Singly or Combined. *Brit. med. J.* ii. 74.

31 BUXTON D.W. (1914) *Anaesthetics*. London: Lewis. 5th ed. p. 173.

32 NUNN J.F. (1968) The Evolution of Atmospheric Oxygen. The Joseph Clover Lecture. *Ann. Roy. Coll. Surg.* **43**. 200–217.

33 HEWITT F.W. (1893) *Anaesthetics and their Administration*. London: Griffin. p. 115.

34 BERT P. (1880) Anésthèsie par le protoxyde d'azote employé sous tension. *Comptes Rendus de la Societé de Biologie.* Tom v. 152.

35 HILLISCHER H.T. (1886) Ueber die allgemeine Verwend barkeit der lustgas—sauerstoffnarkosin in der Chirugie. (Paper to 59th meeting of German Natural Philosophers and Physicians. Berlin, 21 Sept 1886). *Oesterreichisch-Ungarische Kerteljahrsschrift fur Zahnheilkunde,* **2**. 343.

36 WITZEL A. (1889) *Deutsche Zahnkeilunde in Vortragen.* Wein.

37 WOOD H.C. (1893) On the Action of Nitrous Oxid and of the mixture of Nitrous Oxid and Oxygen. *Dental Cosmos.* **35**. 349.

38 HEWITT F.W. (1897) *The Administration of Nitrous Oxide and Oxygen for dental operations.* London: Ash. p. 15.

39 HEWITT F.W. (1894). Further observations on the use of Oxygen with Nitrous Oxide. *J. Brit. Dent. Ass.* **15**. 380–387.

40 DUNCUM B. (1947) *op. cit.* p. 484.

41 All quotations from Hewitt F.W. (1897) *op. cit.* chapters *iv. v. vi. passim.*

42 BOYLE H.E.G. (1907) *Practical Anaesthetics.* London: Hodder & Stoughton. p. 47.

43 BUXTON D.W. (1907) *Anaesthetics.* London: Lewis. 4th ed. p. 105.

44 GARDNER, H. BELLAMY (1916) *Manual of Surgical Anaesthesia.* London: Macmillan. 2nd ed. p. 100.

45 *A Century of Service to Dentistry, 1844–1944.* (1944) S.S.White Dental Manufacturing Company. Philadelphia.

46 *Anaesthesia by Nitrous Oxide and Oxygen Combined* (1903) The S.S.White Dental Manufacturing Company. Philadelphia.

47 *The Clark New Model Gas Apparatus* (1915) The Dental Speciality Co.

48 KING A.C. (1946) The Evolution of Anaesthetic Apparatus. *Brit. med. Bull.* **4**. 136.

49 KING A.C. (1949) [Early Anaesthetic Apparatus.] *Trans. Inst. Brit. Surg. Tech.* **6**. 1.

50 HEIDBRINK J.A. (1957) Memoirs. *Newsmonthly of the American Dental Society of Anesthesiology.* March–May 1957. 1–12.

51 HEIDBRINK J.A. (1957) *ibid.* p. 5.

52 HEIDBRINK J.A. (1957) *ibid.* p. 10.

53 FAULCONER A. and KEYS T.E. (1965) *Foundations of Anesthesiology.* Charles Thomas. Springfield. Vol. 2. p. 746.

54 GWATHMEY J.T. (1913a) Oil-Ether Anesthesia. *N.Y. Med.J.* **98**. 1101.

55 GWATHMEY J.T. (1913b) Oil-Ether Anesthesia. *Lancet.* ii. 1756.

56 BOYLE H.E.G. (1917) Experiences in the Use of Nitrous Oxide and Oxygen with rebreathing in Military Surgery. *Brit. Med.J.* ii. 653.

57 JACKSON D.E. (1915) A New Method for the Production of General Analgesia and Anaesthesia. *J. Lab. Clin. Med.* **1**. 1.

58 COTTON F.J. and BOOTHBY W.M. (1912) Nitrous Oxide-Oxygen-Ether anaesthesia: notes on administration: a perfected apparatus. *Surgery, Gynaecology and Obstetrics.* **15**. 281.

59 GWATHMEY J.T. (1914) *Anesthesia.* New York: Appleton. p. 171.

60 KAYE G., ORTON R.H., RENTON D.G. (1946) *Anaesthetic Methods.* Melbourne: Ramsay. p. 291.

61 MARSHALL G. (1917a)
Anaesthetics for Men with
Wounds of the Abdomen.
Lancet. **i**. 640.

62 MARSHALL G. (1917a) *ibid*.

63 MARSHALL G. (1917b) The
Administration of Anaesthetics
at the Front. *Brit. Med. J*. **i**.
722.

64 Ross G. (1919) *Anaesthetics*.
Edinburgh: Livingstone. p. 70.

65 BOYLE H.E.G. (1919a) Nitrous
Oxide-Oxygen-Ether Outfit.
Lancet. **i**. 226.

66 MARSHALL G. (1920) Two
types of portable Gas-oxygen
Apparatus. *Proc. Roy. Soc. Med*.
13. 1. (*Anaesth. Sect*.) p. 18.

67 Obituary notice: (1941)
H.E.G.Boyle. *Lancet*. **ii**. 546.

68 HADFIELD C.J. (1950).
H.Edmund G.Boyle. *Brit. J*.
Anaesth. **22**. 107.

69 BUXTON D.W. (1914)
Anaesthetics. London: Lewis.
5th ed. p. 197.

70 BOYLE H.E.G. (1919a) *op. cit*.
p. 226

71 BOYLE H.E.G. (1919b) Nitrous-
oxide-oxygen-ether outfit. *Brit*.
med. J. **i**. 159.

72 BOYLE H.E.G. (1918) Nitrous-
oxide-oxygen-ether outfit. *Proc*.
Roy. Soc. Med. **11**. 1. (*Anaesth*.
Sect.). p. 30.

73 LEE J.A. and ATKINSON R.S.
(1973) *Synopsis of Anaesthesia*.
Bristol: Wright. 7th ed.
p. 132–133.

74 SHIPWAY F.E. (1920)
Apparatus for Nitrous Oxide,
Oxygen and Ether. *Proc. Roy*.

Soc. Med. **13**. 1. (*Anaesth*.
Sect.). p. 20.

75 Obituary notices: (1955)
H.N.Webber. *Anaesthesia*. **10**.
207. *Brit. med. J*. **i**. 172.

76 ROOD F.S. and WEBBER H.N.
(1930) *Anaesthesia and
Anaesthetics*. London: Cassell.

77 BOURNE, WESLEY (1955)
Mysterious Waters to Guard.
Oxford: Blackwell. p. 78.

78 GWATHMEY J.T. (1925)
Anesthesia. New York:
Macmillan. 2nd ed. p. 722.

79 MCKESSON E.I. (1920)
Advances in pure Nitrous
Oxide-Oxygen Anaesthesia.
Amer. J. Surg. **34**. 10.

80 SYKES W.S. (1935) Anaesthesia,
its present and future. *Brit. J*.
Anaesth. **13**. 51.

81 MCKESSON E.I. (1926a) Gas-
and-oxygen Anesthesia in
Abdominal Surgery: and
'Secondary Saturation' *Proc.
Roy. Soc. Med*. **19**. 57–64.

82 MCKESSON E.I. (1911) Nitrous
oxide-oxygen Anaesthesia, with
a description of a new
apparatus. *Surgery, Gynec.
Obst*. **13**. 456–62.

83 HENDERSON Y. (1925)
Respiration in Anaesthesia:
Control by Carbon Dioxide.
Brit. med. J. **ii**. 1170–1175.

84 MCKESSON E.I. (1926b) Some
Physical Factors in the
Administration of Gaseous
Anaesthetics. *Brit. med. J*. **ii**.
1113–1117.

85 *McKesson Nargraf for General
Anaesthesia*. (1930). McKesson
Appliance Co. Toledo. pub. by

A.Charles King, Ltd., London.
(figs. 3.61., 3.67).

86 MENNELL Z. (1935) The Second
Embley Lecture. *Brit. J.
Anaesth*. **13**. 18.

87 NAINBY-LUXMOORE R.C. (1967)
Some hazards of dental gas
machines. *Anaesthesia*. **22**. 545.

88 *The Walton* **2** *Instruction
Pamphlet*. (1938). British
Oxygen Co. Ltd.

89 CONNELL K. (1913). A new
ether vaporiser. *Journal of
American Medical Association*.
60. 892.

90 BICKHAM W.S. (1924) *Operative
Surgery*. Philadelphia. Saunders.
Vol. I. p. 157.

91 Obituary notice: (1941) Karl
Connell. *Newsletter of the
American Society of
Anesthetists*. IV. (11). p. 4.

ILLUSTRATIONS

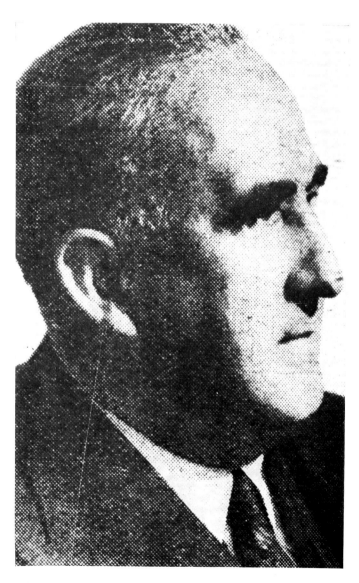

FIG. 4.1. SIR ROBERT ERNEST
KELLY, 1879–1944.
From *Lancet*, 1944, **ii**, 740.
obituary notice.

CKC 23: KELLY INTRATRACHEAL ETHER APPARATUS 1912 as modified by Shipway

This apparatus was labelled by King as *Kelly's Intratracheal Ether Apparatus* of 1912, and his attribution was accepted for the published inventory[1]. Upon closer investigation however, it has been found that Francis Shipway (later Sir Francis) modified an earlier model designed by Robert Kelly (later Sir Robert). Comparative details will be given below.

Robert Ernest Kelly (Fig. 4.1), 1879–1944, was Liverpool born and bred, and was one of the first medical graduates of the University of Liverpool when it was constituted[2, 3], qualifying in 1901. On retiring from the Chair of Surgery at his old University he was knighted in 1939. His range of surgical interest was wide, though its main appeal seems to have been in orthopaedics and brain surgery. As a good and hospitable Liverpudlian, Kelly welcomed visiting Americans passing through the city, and was always alive to the new ideas which they brought with them.

Thus in 1912 Kelly introduced the method of intratracheal insufflation of ether which had been inaugurated in 1909 by Samuel Meltzer and John Auer, then working at the Rockefeller Institute[4]. These investigators discovered that respiration can be carried on in the curarized animal by continuous inflation of the lungs without any normal or artificial rhythmical respiratory movements. This they achieved *either* by a tube—two-thirds of the tracheal diameter—passing through a tracheostomy to the tracheal bifurcation *or* by the use of two tubes inserted through separate tracheal openings, *or* by a catheter passed through an O'Dwyer laryngeal tube inserted through the mouth. In each case the removal

of carbon dioxide took place by a different path from that through which air was insufflated. Meltzer and Auer stated 'The following three points are the essential factors in the success of our method. (1) the lungs are kept in a continuous inspiratory state of distension which facilitates the exchange of the gases. (2) the fresh air reaches the lowest part of the trachea (3) the air escapes by another path (although also through the trachea) than the one by which it enters. Under these conditions the supply of oxygen and removal of carbon dioxide takes place apparently in physiological fashion without the aid of any rhythmic antagonistic movements.'[5]

It may be noted that they saw the effects of increasing intrathoracic pressure (if the tube was too large, or tied tightly into the trachea). Cyanosis of the lungs ensued, and was relieved by disconnecting the tube from the pressure bottle for two seconds, giving a momentary collapse of the lungs. They were too early to appreciate the circulatory significance of this manoeuvre. It is interesting too that they quoted two forerunners of their method; firstly the experiment of Robert Hook in 1667, in sustaining the life of a thoracotomized dog whose lungs had been punctured in various places, by continuous inflation of the lungs: and secondly Nagel's (1900) method of maintaining the respiration of curarized pigeons by sending a continuous stream of air through the humerus which in these birds is connected with the air sacs. In this case the air escaped through the trachea, but in both instances, as in the case of Meltzer and Auer's experiment, by a separate path from that through which it had entered the lungs.

The method of Meltzer and Auer rapidly passed into anaesthesia, being developed in particular by C.A.Elsberg, Frederick Cotton and Chevalier Jackson in America, and later by Ivan Magill and

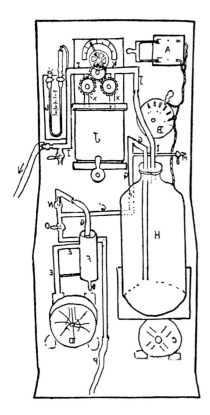

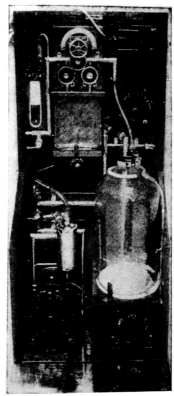

FIG. 4.2. ELSBERG INTRATRACHEAL APPARATUS, for insufflation of ether. An electric motor supplies a flow of air, and the three cogwheel control was borrowed by both Shipway and Kelly.
From Buxton,D.W. (1914). *Anaesthetics*. London: Lewis, p. 191.

Stanley Rowbotham in England.

It is not now known who inspired Robert Kelly to produce the first insufflation apparatus in England, but in 1912 he described[6] a simplified version of Elsberg's design which had been published in 1911[7], (Fig. 4.2).

Kelly wrote enthusiastically of the method, describing it as a method both of respiration and of anaesthetization and pointing to its value for the future development of thoracic surgery.

Both Elsberg and Kelly used an electric motor and pump to supply a flow of air, and Elsberg's three wheel control is a characteristic also of the Kelly version (Fig. 4.3) and of the Shipway modification (Fig. 4.4).

The pressure was maintained at between 10 and 30mm mercury 'sufficient' Kelly remarks 'to inflate the lungs and to maintain efficient oxygenation of

FIG. 4.3. KELLY INTRATRACHEAL
ETHER INSUFFLATOR, 1912.
The air flow was supplied by
electric motor and the air-ether
mixture heated by passing through
a coil in a water bath. The

intratracheal insufflation catheter is
shown (22 French gauge = 5mm
internal diameter).
From Buxton,D.W. (1914). *ibid.*
p. 194.

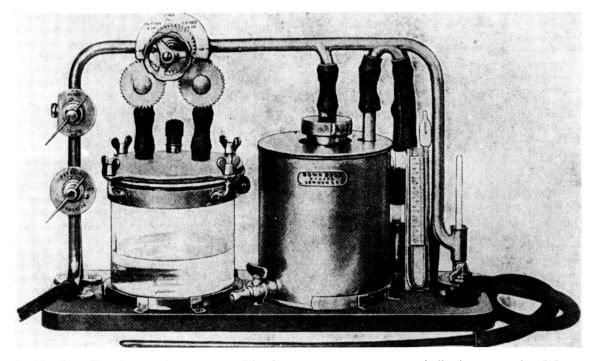

the blood'. A French 22 catheter was used in the adult, passed under direct vision to the bifurcation of the trachea, using Chevalier Jackson's laryngoscope.

From the blower, air passed through two tap controls, the upper of which has a side tube for oxygen, to the mixing device controlled by the cogwheel system; the main wheel is marked 'air/½ ether ½ air/ full', according to the wheel setting. A side tube leads outwards at this point to a mercury blow-off safety-valve. From the control, the air may be passed wholly or in part into the large glass ether bottle down a wide-bore tube. The ether/air mixture then passes through a metal coil in a hot water bath (a

mercury manometer indicating pressure) and thence to the patient via a long rubber tube and the intratracheal catheter, of 22 French gauge, which is about one quarter of the tracheal diameter (see Figs. 4.3, 4.4). Fig. 4.3 is of the original Kelly pattern, the differences being of detail only. The main improvement in the Shipway version (Fig. 4.5) probably consisted of the longer ether tube, providing a higher percentage of ether vapour. Both versions have a hot water bath with a coil. Warm ether was a particular feature of this period in anaesthesia, and one favoured especially by Sir Francis Shipway.

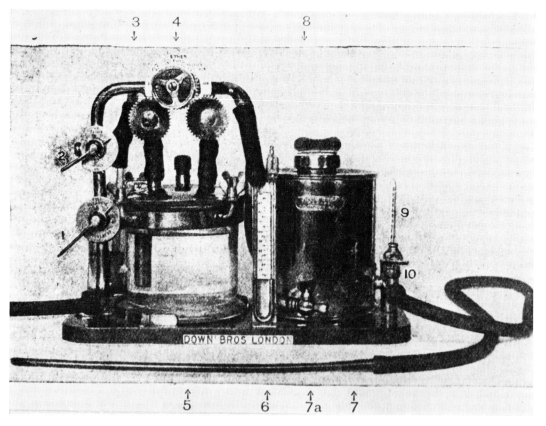

CKC 25, 26: SHIPWAY WARM ETHER and CHLOROFORM APPARATUS, for INTRATRACHEAL INSUFFLATION 1916

Francis Edward Shipway, (Fig. 4.6) 1875–1968, honorary anaesthetist to Guy's Hospital from 1908 to 1938, was one of the leaders of the speciality, whose pronouncements and papers appeared regularly in the journals and proceedings of societies.

In 1925–26 he was President of the Section of Anaesthetics of the Royal Society of Medicine, and in the same year he achieved popular notice as anaesthetist to King George V when the monarch had a rib resection performed for an empyema. The honour of knighthood followed[8].

Shipway is best known for the apparatus here described, which served anaesthetists as a readily portable alternative both to the Clover ether inhaler (p. 14) and to the Junker's chloroform apparatus

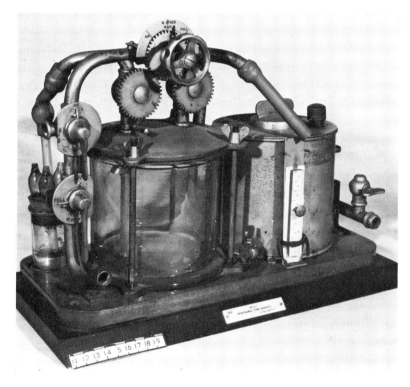

FIG. 4.5. SHIPWAY'S
MODIFICATION
of Kelly's intratracheal ether
insufflator.
(Cf. Fig. 4.4).
CKC 23

(p. 68) of which he made use. Shipway's design was based on his oft repeated contention that warm anaesthetic vapours are advantageous to the patient[9, 10].

Earlier anaesthetists such as Snow and Clover had adopted measures to ensure warming of the ether containers in their various pieces of apparatus; some have therefore asserted that this was done in recognition of the advantage to the patient: in fact, as Shipway pointed out[9], a study of the apparatus and of the original articles shows that the efforts to warm the vaporizer were made to assist the

administrator by avoiding over-cooling, rather than to benefit the patient. Shipway was further influenced by some American anaesthetists, notably Gwathmey, who had performed a large number of experimental observations upon the temperature and effects of cooling in anaesthetized dogs[11]. Gwathmey began this paper with a reference to Seelig of St Louis[12], who had other views, and who concluded that 'despite the fact that ether vapour was driven through a temperature approximating 100°C. it radiated its acquired heat so rapidly that at a distance of one metre from the source of

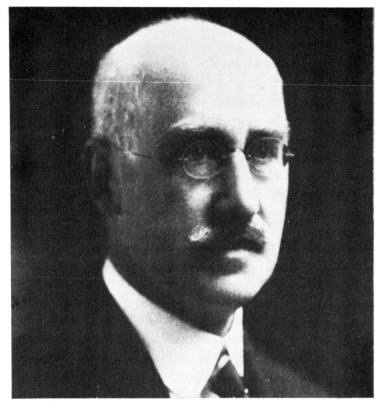

FIG. 4.6. SIR FRANCIS SHIPWAY,
K.C.V.O., 1875–1968.
Anaesthetist to Guy's Hospital.
From *British Medical Journal* (1968)
iv, 649, obituary notice.

heat it had practically assumed room temperature'. This is probably near the truth. Gwathmey however, repeated these experiments with different results and then went on to perform animal experiments showing, for example, that chloroform at blood temperature is three times as safe as chloroform at room temperature, based on the times taken to kill his animals. Similar results were claimed using nitrous oxide/oxygen, and ether. Gwathmey also maintained that animals recovered more rapidly after the use of warmed vapours, and even suggested that in human beings, 'it may be stated that by applying hot towels to the patient's face, or aerating the lungs with hot air toward the close of any anaesthesia, the patient is brought out quickly, and this procedure aids considerably in modifying the unpleasant after effects'[11].

Shipway took up these ideas with enthusiasm, and condemned the use of 'open ether', which caused lowering of the temperature of the inhaled air. He

FIG. 4.7. SHIPWAY WARM ETHER/
CHLOROFORM INTRATRACHEAL
APPARATUS, 1916.
The ether bottle carries a control
tap; chloroform is vaporized from a
Junker's bottle; neither ether nor
chloroform percentages can be
controlled. The vacuum flask
contains a coiled tube in hot water,
which allegedly warms the vapours
before delivery to the patient.
(Cf. Fig. 4.8).
CKC 25

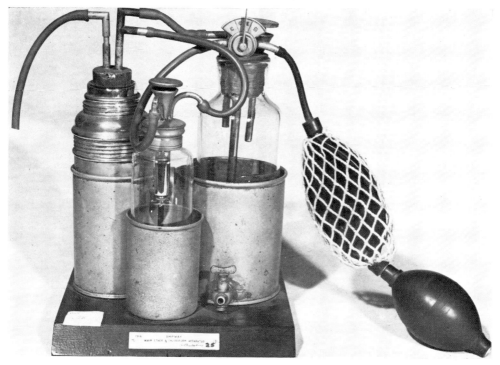

maintained that 'warm vapours are more pleasant to inhale and are more readily absorbed by the blood'[9], and quoted Teter, another American protagonist of warm vapours, to the effect that, 'of 40 women who inhaled nitrous oxide (90°F) many were unconscious after two or three breaths, whilst if cold nitrous oxide were given the majority were conscious up to the tenth, or even the twentieth, breath'[13]. Shipway also showed an experimental temperature table in which, for example, at a room temperature of 68°F and water temperature 116°, ether vapour at the end of a 30 in (76.5cm) rubber tube, issued at 86°F. A recent experiment under-

taken by the writer has failed to confirm these figures. Shipway also claimed fewer post-operative lung complications, but there seems no doubt that much of the improvement was due to the use of the intratracheal catheter, which was at that time a technique greatly used by the more able anaesthetist, and one which was facilitated by the use of the Shipway apparatus.

The apparatus itself consisted of a large capacity hand bellows, an ether bottle, a chloroform bottle, (Junker's pattern) and a vacuum bottle as a warming flask (CKC 25, Fig. 4.7). The tubing was arranged to pass the vapours through these bottles and a two

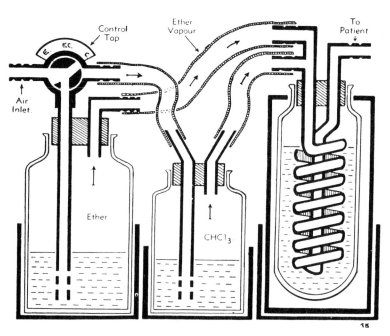

FIG. 4.8. SHIPWAY APPARATUS.
Diagram from Kaye,G., Orton,
R.H. and Renton,D.C. (1946)
Anaesthetic Methods. Melbourne:
Ramsay, p. 187.

way tap on the ether bottle allowed the air to be blown through either or both the anaesthetic liquids. (Fig. 4.8). The more refined version dispensed with the vacuum flask and substituted a hot water canister through which chloroform vapour was blown from the bottle K, (Fig. 4.9) while ether was vaporized from the container B via drip feed D, before passing to the intratracheal catheter. A mercury manometer and thermometer were added, and the specimen in the collection (CKC 26) is carried in a padded box. It cost £5.8.0d at Messrs. Mayer in 1925 (Fig. 4.10).

Shipway's apparatus was without doubt a useful and satisfactory method of *insufflating* chloroform and/or ether vapours down an intratracheal catheter.

At a meeting of the Section of Anaesthetists of the Royal Society of Medicine on 4 February, 1921, Dr H.J.Shirley being in the chair, Rowbotham and Magill read their famous paper on anaesthesia for facial plastic surgery. In the discussion which followed 'Dr. Shipway said that there could be no doubt that intratracheal ether was much superior to the older methods of anaesthesia for operations on the face. . . . He was glad Mr Rowbotham and Mr Magill had condemned the use of his warm ether apparatus as a *draw-over* inhaler. It was never intended to be used in that way, as the lumen of the tubes was much too small and the dead-space was considerable'[14]. No special mention was made by any speaker of the need for warm ether vapour,

(See Fig. 4.10).
From Ross and Fairlie. (1929)
Handbook of Anaesthetics.
Edinburgh: Livingstone.

FIG. 4.10. SHIPWAY WARM ETHER/
CHLOROFORM APPARATUS
CKC 26

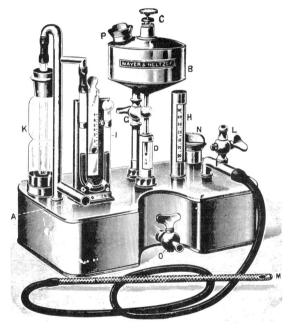

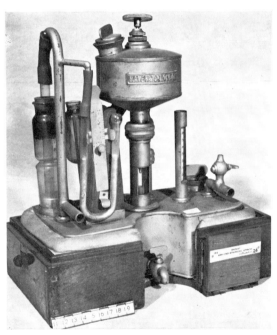

though the use of the Shipway insufflator implied this. We shall see that Magill also introduced an apparatus which produced warm ether (CKC 34, p. 190).

CKC 33: ROWBOTHAM SIDCUP INTRATRACHEAL APPARATUS 1921

Dr Edgar Stanley Rowbotham (b. 1890) (Fig. 4.11), now lives in retirement in Madeira following long attachment to Charing Cross Hospital. We shall discuss again below the work of Rowbotham and Magill at the Queen's Hospital for Facio-Maxillary Injuries at Sidcup in the years immediately after the

Great War.

In their original paper[15] they described their experiences in 3,000 cases and their techniques are worth closer enquiry. They premedicated patients with atropine gr 1/50 (1.2mg), and wrote, 'one of us administers 1/6 gr (10mg) of morphine unless specially contraindicated, whilst the other gives 1/4 gr (15mg) in only those cases in which gas and oxygen are to be given.' The difficulties encountered derived from the extreme intolerance of the patients to anaesthetics, especially to multiple administrations of ether, and in particular from those of maintaining the airway. They also found that patients were far more fearful of the anaesthetic than of the operation, remarking that 'flying officers who had a

FIG. 4.11. DR E.S. ROWBOTHAM,
Charing Cross and Royal Free
Hospitals.

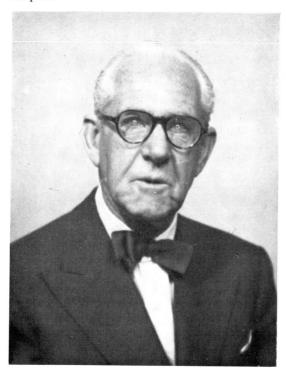

FIG. 4.11. DR E.S. ROWBOTHAM,
Charing Cross and Royal Free
Hospitals.

crash seem to be particularly nervous, some of them
going through their fall again whilst going under.'
The administration was either by Shipway's three
bottle warm ether apparatus (CKC 25, p. 185) using
a Hewitt's or Phillip's airway, or by an angle-piece
(Rowbotham's) and funnel with wide-bore tube, or
by intratracheal insufflation of nitrous oxide-oxygen-
ether. The latter is given as the method of choice,
being used in nine out of ten cases. Generally a

double tube system was used but it is interesting to
notice that the second tube was only passed 'almost
as far as the glottis' and not through it.

Another technique described in this important
and fascinating paper is that of nitrous oxide
analgesia combined with morphine premedication
and local infiltration of 1 per cent novocaine and
adrenalin 1 in 1000, 3 drops to the ounce (= 27
cu ml), a method similar to that of Crile.

This paper adumbrates the use of wide-bore
endotracheal tubes in the remark 'in one or two
cases we have passed a stout rubber tube through
the glottis by direct vision and connected it with the
wide tube and gas bag with satisfactory results.' In
the discussion which followed W.J.McCardie of
Birmingham remarked 'in nasal intubation it was
important that the tubes should have as large a
lumen as possible,' though he referred only to gum
elastic catheters.

'Mr. Rowbotham (in reply) said that in passing
the catheter through the nose, it did sometimes
happen that it could be pushed straight on into the
trachea, without any other manipulation being
required, but in these cases experience had shown
the need for some other more certain means of
guiding it. . . . Shaping the tube at its end to a
point, smearing it with Vaseline, and gradual and
gentle dilatation, starting with a very small tube,
seemed to be the main points.'

Laryngoscopes and the introduction hooks and
forceps (now universally known as Magill's) were
shown.

Rowbotham originally described 'blind' nasal
intubation with a catheter[16] but it will be
appropriate at this point to consider a little further
the origins of the wide-bore endotracheal tube.
Though this is indelibly associated with the name of
Magill, no apology need be made for its inclusion in

a section devoted to Rowbotham, the two names being so much interwoven in this interesting period of anaesthetic history.

Sir Ivan Magill has told the present author that in 1920 Sir Harold Gillies had a patient with a nasal injury who refused chloroform or ether. Magill decided to pass nitrous oxide and oxygen down a large-bore tube rather than a catheter. After secondary saturation with nitrous oxide (see p. 156) the patient was intubated with a piece of rubber tubing cut off a Boyle's machine and bevelled. Sir Ivan remarked that 'she was a bit blue' but all went well.

In spite of this successful debut, insufflation continued to be used by what Sir Ivan described as the true process, that is 'the abolition of spontaneous respiration by a high flow of gases through two catheters lying in the trachea, and passed either through the nose or mouth.' In 1927 Magill was still describing this technique for dental work[17], but on 7 February 1930, again at the Royal Society of Medicine, he said 'continuous high pressure insufflation as described by Meltzer and Auer, is unnecessary for most thoracic operations. . . . I prefer to insufflate at as low a pressure as is sufficient to abolish the dead space in the trachea and to control expiration directly. This can be done by means of a wide-bore return tube, or by using only one wide-bore tube and an adjustable expiratory valve'[18].

At the same time, Magill developed his blind nasal intubation technique, and H.W. Featherstone remarked 'Dr Magill's special rubber-intratracheal tube for blind intubation through the nose excited much interest and admiration' (in Canada)[19].

It is evident that to these great anaesthetists Magill and Rowbotham, the actual machinery mattered little. It was the man and the method which counted, and improvisation was the order, as is shown by Magill's use of a piece of tubing from a Boyle's machine for wide-bore intubation.

Rowbotham described wide-bore intubation in a lecture given at the Cancer Hospital in 1926[20]. After describing insufflation methods, both by single and double catheter, he said 'It occurred to me that if one could pass a single tube of adequate size through the mouth (or nose) and into the trachea, and allow the patient to breathe backwards and forwards through it, a state of things much more akin to that which occurs during natural respiration would be achieved. Moreover, the first part of the respiratory passages would be just as well cut out: and providing that the tube were sufficiently large to fill the glottic opening, there would be no danger of blood entering the trachea. This was found to be no more difficult than passing the smaller return airway for use with a catheter.'

This piece of apparatus designed by Rowbotham, and now in the King Collection (No. 33), may almost be counted as an aberration, and in its incomplete state it is not easy to see its method of use.

It consists of a rectangular tin warm water box (Fig. 4.12) through which a coiled tube circulates. Through the tube, air, oxygen or nitrous oxide could be pumped, to pick up ether vapour from a drip fitting, now incomplete, before passing to the patient's endotracheal catheter. So heartily was the warm ether concept embraced at this time (c. 1920) that the box also had a large bore tube driven through it, in which an electric light bulb could be placed. There are also a rubber diaphragm valve and an air-opening, the uses of which are not now readily understood. This apparatus was an experiment of Dr Rowbotham's, far surpassed by his other contributions to endotracheal anaesthesia.

FIG. 4.13. SIR IVAN WHITESIDE
MAGILL K.C.V.O.

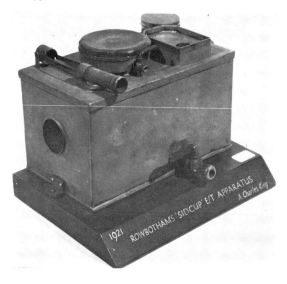

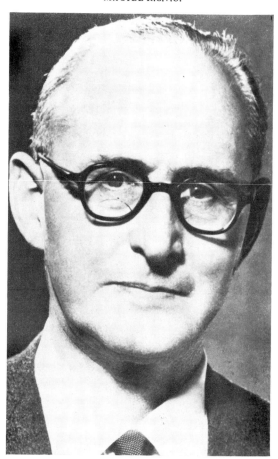

CKC 34: MAGILL INTRATRACHEAL APPARATUS 1921

Sir Ivan Magill, (Fig. 4.13) was born at Larne in Northern Ireland in 1888, and is known to all as the doyen of British anaesthetists, and indeed, of the world. As a captain in the Royal Army Medical Corps with the Expeditionary Forces to France in the Great War, and later at the Queens Hospital for Maxillo-Facial Injuries at Sidcup, he and Dr Rowbotham did pioneer work in the use of intratracheal insufflation and later, endotracheal anaesthesia as we now recognize it. Laryngoscopes, forceps, tubes and connectors were designed by them and the majority, in world wide use, bear Magill's name.

The original paper describing the work at Sidcup was given to the Section of Anaesthetics of the Royal Society of Medicine on 4 February 1921[21]. The Magill intratracheal apparatus was not specifically mentioned in this paper, which described the use of a funnel apparatus for 'draw-over' anaesthesia, the use of the Shipway warm ether apparatus and lastly and most importantly, the intratracheal insufflation of nitrous oxide, oxygen and ether. This paper has already been discussed in detail above (p. 187).

Two months later, a short paper in the *Lancet* fully described the present 'blow-over' apparatus[22]. The Charles King Collection specimen is identical with that shown in the *Lancet* paper (Figs. 4.14, 4.15), with the minor exception that it has a U-tube mercury manometer in place of the more expensive, but more portable, dial manometer. The main

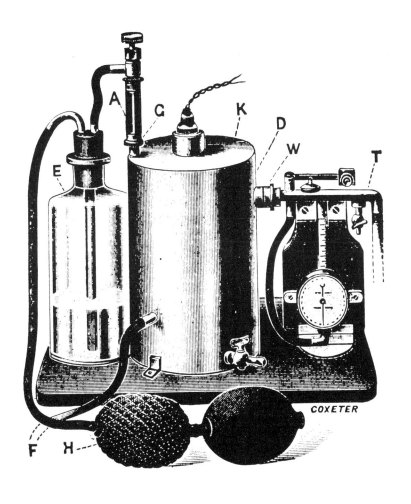

A
G
K
D
W
E
T
COXETER
F
H

FIG. 4.14. MAGILL INTRATRACHEAL INSUFFLATION APPARATUS, 1921.

Two pressure sources are used. The hand bellows forces ether over to the drip-feed at A. In the heated vaporizer K, the vapour is picked up under pressure from a foot pump (or air cylinder), entering the system through tube F. The tube T passes the ether-air mixture to a narrow-bore intratracheal gum-elastic catheter.

From Magill, I.W. (1921) A Portable Apparatus for Tracheal Insufflation. *Lancet*, **i**, 918.

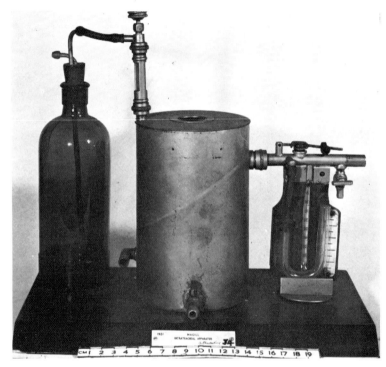

FIG. 4.15. MAGILL
INTRATRACHEAL INSUFFLATION
APPARATUS, 1921.
(Cf. Fig. 4.14).
CKC 34

feature is the heating chamber D, which comprises an outer cylinder 6 in (15cm) by 4 in (10.5cm), and an inner cylinder 4 in (10.5cm) by 3 in (7cm), the intervening space forming a closed air chamber, into which ether is dripped from the needle valve sight feed (A), after being forced over under low pressure by a hand pump from the ether bottle (E). Air from a foot pump or compressed air cylinder enters the lower part of the air chamber at (F), passes around the inner cylinder and leaves by the tube (W), carrying vaporized ether to the patient via tube (T). The safety-valve manometer and thermometer are mounted on a wooden support connected with the tube (T). The air chamber is heated by hot water, or as in the diagram and in no. 34 by an electric light bulb. This piece of apparatus, and its lucid descrip-

tion in his paper, show the genius of Sir Ivan Magill for practical ideas, even though such ideas were rapidly outmoded, mainly by his own continuing work.

CKC 38: MAGILL INTRATRACHEAL APPARATUS 1927

This apparatus (Figs. 4.16, 4.17) was described by Magill[23] as 'a fusion into one composite unit of an endotracheal ether insufflation apparatus and a nitrous oxide and oxygen apparatus.' Both had been described in the *Lancet*, in 1921[24] and 1923[25], and the first of these is No. 34 in the King Collection (p. 190.) The second is shown from Magill's descrip-

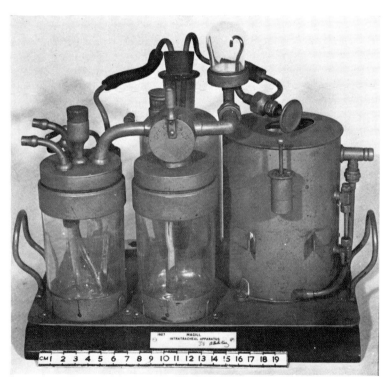

tion (Fig. 4.18). A new feature of this was described by Magill: 'The N_2O inlet to the water sight feed bottle (S.) is made partly of metal and partly of glass, the metal part having a hole above the water-level equal to the calibre of the tube itself. When the N_2O is turned on the level of the water in the glass-tube is depressed, such level indicating regularity of flow. A depression of $\frac{3}{4}$ in represents approximately a flow of 120 gallons of N_2O per hour. The oblique construction of the oxygen tube (O) enables the bubbles to be plainly seen. . . . Two 'holes' of oxygen with a depression of $\frac{3}{4}$ in. in the N_2O tube represents 10 per cent of oxygen'[25].

The warmed ether intracheal apparatus of 1921 (No. 34, Fig. 4.15) was improved by altering the ether drop feed 'to the shape of a dome which can be easily seen from any angle'[23]. An extra bottle was added for ether, pressure being supplied by hand bellows, as in the 1921 apparatus, to supply ether to the dome where it was vaporized, to be mixed with the incoming nitrous oxide and oxygen (perhaps with chloroform or chloroform-ether), before passing to the heating chamber (Fig. 4.17). The manufacturers were Down Bros.

FIG. 4.17. THE SAME APPARATUS
as described by Sir Ivan Magill in
Lancet (1927) **ii**, 396. (See Fig. 4.16)

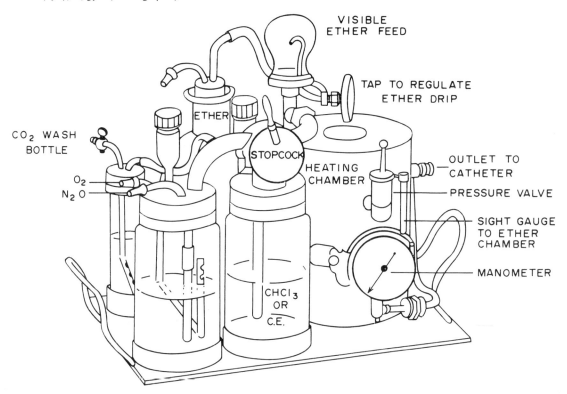

CKC 43: MAGILL ENDOTRACHEAL APPARATUS 1932

An artificial distinction appears to have been created by the use of the words 'intratracheal' and 'endotracheal'. In the context of the passage of anaesthetic vapours, there can be no semantic difference between the two words, whatever the etymological difference, but it is convenient to follow the original precedent, and to use 'intratracheal' where insufflation by catheter is implied, and 'endotracheal' where the modern type of wide-bore tube is used. The same vaporizing apparatus could be used for either, but, as in the present case, the apparatus seems to have been used for 'endotracheal' use and is so described, though a metal label merely calls it 'Dr Ivan Magill's Apparatus, Reg. Design No. 771428, A.Charles King Limited, London.'

This apparatus (Fig. 4.19) is an improved and neater version of No. 38 and so is an amalgam of those of 1921 and 1923 with the addition of flowmeters. This is the earliest piece of apparatus in the King

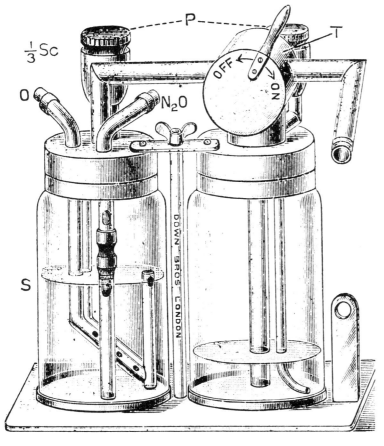

FIG. 4.18. MAGILL NITROUS
OXIDE-OXYGEN-ETHER
APPARATUS OF 1923.
It was incorporated with the
intratracheal apparatus of 1921
(Fig. 4.15) to form the machine
(Fig. 4.17), of 1927.
From *Lancet*, 1923, **ii**, 228.

Collection to employ dry flowmeters, though the collection possesses a pair of similar coupled Siebe-Gorman flowmeters (No. 40) used by Dr Magill in 1928. In the present case, two flowmeters, graduated to 20 litres for nitrous oxide, and 10 litres for oxygen, pass the gases to a cross tube which goes to a chloroform bottle and thence to a vertical tube into which liquid ether may be dropped via a curved tube and dome, as in No. 38. A bypass (with tap) from the oxygen side can be used to pass the gas into the ether container on which the flowmeters are mounted. Thence liquid ether is driven to the drip chamber. The mixed gases then move to a warming chamber (with manometer and safety-valve) mounted over a

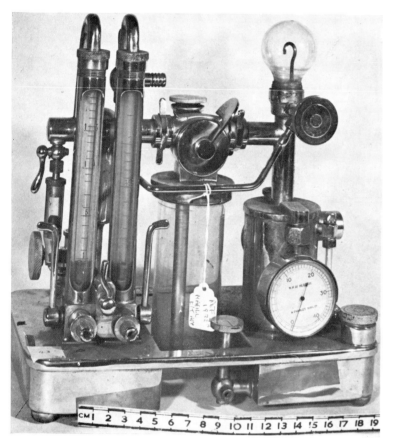

FIG. 4.19. MAGILL
ENDOTRACHEAL APPARATUS,
1932.
This apparatus is an improved
version of that of 1927. (p. 192
No. 38). To the left, below, is the
ether container, and to the right,
the warm water container. The
glass bottle contained chloroform
and the metal cylinder behind the
manometer is for mixing and
warming the gases and vapours.
The flowmeters are graduated to
20 litres for nitrous oxide, and 10
litres for oxygen and have separate
control levers. Behind is a carbon
dioxide flow gauge. The wide-bore
outlet is on right. A rebreathing
bag was mounted behind the mixing
chamber.
CKC 43

warm water container before going to the patient
through a tube of $\frac{1}{2}$ in (1.3cm) diameter. Compared
to the outlet tubes on the 'intratracheal' apparatus,
this is a relatively wide bore. At the rear of the
warming chamber is a very wide tube 1.4 in (3.5cm)
on which a rebreathing bag was mounted (not
present in example shown). This and the wide-
bore outlet are the only concessions to the 'endotracheal' concept.

A sparklet attachment is fitted for carbon dioxide,
and the whole is neat, practical and portable with
such refinements as visible level indicators on the
ether warm water containers and a small (uncalibra-
ted) flowgauge (a cork with a wire) for carbon dioxide.

No published description of the apparatus has
been found.

FIG. 4.20. PHILLIPS 'AUTOMATIC'
ETHER VAPORIZER. C. 1925.
The small diameter inlet and outlet
tubes are shown. The interior
channels are even more minute.
CKC 36

CKC 36: PHILLIPS 'AUTOMATIC' ETHER VAPORIZER *c.* 1925

The name of Hugh Richard Phillips, M.D., Edinburgh (1874–1932) first appears in the Annual Reports of the Italian Hospital of London as a 'chloroformist' in 1902. He was awarded the title *Cavaliera* in 1920 and remained on the staff of the hospital until 1931[26], being also for ten years on the staff of the Great Ormond Street Hospital for Sick Children. His obituary notices[27] speak of his 'mighty physique', his apparatus was always 'perfectly adjusted', and he 'had a peculiar skill in managing difficult children and very old people.' His papers include those on open ether and oxygen; and on anaesthesia for tonsillectomy, for which he advocated chloroform and oxygen,[28]: Phillips also described anaesthesia for two patients with a patent ductus arteriosus, one in childbirth and one for dental extraction, using Hewitt's nitrous oxide/oxygen apparatus for the first, and warmed oxygen/chloroform for the second patient[29], probably employing the method which he described in 1918 as a three-bottle apparatus for oxygen-chloroform-ether[30]. This does not appear to be connected with the present piece, for which no details have been found. It was described by Charles King as an 'automatic ether' apparatus, and was ascribed by him to *circa* 1925 (Fig. 4.20).

No description has been found in the journals, and the apparatus now consists only of an ether vaporizing bottle of brown glass, marked 'Wellcome Chem. Works.' The neck is fitted with an elaborate metal collar into which screws a cap and dip tube; an inlet tube with a ball valve permits pressure from a hand bulb or oxygen cylinder to pass into the bottle via a tiny passage. Ether liquid is thus forced up the dip-tube, the upper end of which is occluded by a

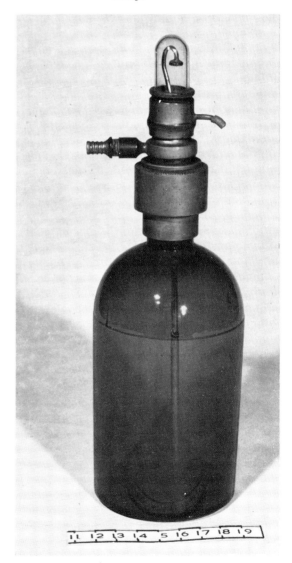

metal pin fixed to an upper collar. If this is rotated on its screw thread, space is allowed for the liquid to pass, through two small holes in the pin, up a curved hollow tube under a glass dome. On being released from this tube the ether presumably vaporizes and passes again through minute passages onwards to the patient. As the apparatus is incomplete it is not possible to state whether any form of bag or other bottle was inserted between the vaporizer and the face mask or intratracheal tube.

The piece is something of an oddity, but appears to have been an attempt to copy the vaporizers of Magill (see No. 43, p. 194) in which the glass dome method was also used. The 'automatic' element of King's ascription was no doubt given since it would be possible by rotating the upper collar, automatically to control within small limits the amount of ether liquid to be vaporized. However, it has proved impossible to make the apparatus perform in this way. Liquid ether appears at the outlet tube!

CKC 42: LEWIS INTRATRACHEAL APPARATUS 1931

Ivor Nicholas Lewis, M.R.C.S., L.R.C.P., D.A., (Eng.) was appointed anaesthetist to St George's Hospital in 1930, and he died two years later in tragic circumstances, at the age of 32. He had already made a mark at St George's, for in addition to developing an extensive practice, he was the first at that hospital to use nembutal; the first to use percaine (nupercaine) for spinal analgesia; the first to give intravenous evipan: and the first to use wide-bore and nasal intubation[31]. He also devised the Lewis portable nitrous oxide-oxygen-ether-chloroform machine. The apparatus was made by Charles King with registered design No 763860, and it was

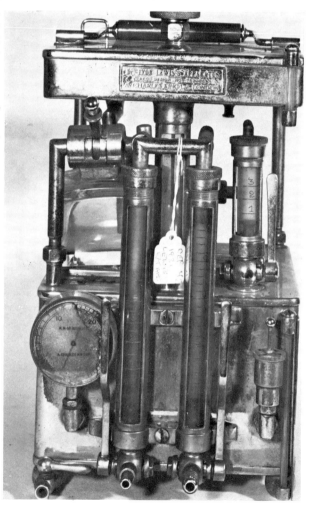

FIG. 4.21. LEWIS INTRATRACHEAL APPARATUS, 1931.
Above, the ether tank with drip-feed control; chloroform bottle to left on top of large water tank with nitrous oxide and oxygen dry flowmeters in front. The outlet to the patient is a narrow-bore tube at rear.
CKC 42

described fully by Lewis in the *Lancet*[32], with a photograph which shows it to have been identical with the present specimen (Fig. 4.21). This bears the number 23. Other examples are known, though its compactness and apparent complexity must have taxed the concentration of the most observant anaesthetist, and it does not appear to have become popular.

Lewis wrote 'The apparatus has been devised to provide the maximum anaesthetic equipment in the minimum of space: the machine is in fact no more than a rearrangement of that designed by Dr Ivan Magill, with the substitution of a gravity feed drip for the ether as used on Shipway's endotracheal (sic) apparatus'[32].

The similarity to Magill's apparatus of 1927 (described on p. 192. Fig. 4.16) is not readily apparent, even when the two examples are examined side by side, but the principles are the same: a nitrous oxide-oxygen-chloroform flow picked up ether vapour from a drip, and, passing through a warmed chamber, was conveyed by narrow-bore outlet (1 cm) tube to the patient. Thus the apparatus was intended for insufflation.

The overall measurements of Lewis's apparatus are $6\frac{1}{2}$ in $\times$ $6\frac{1}{2}$ in $\times$ 11 in (16.5cm $\times$ 16.5cm $\times$ 28cm)* and a remarkable series of tanks and tubes were fitted into this small space.

Nitrous oxide (15 litre) and oxygen (5 litre) flowmeters received the gases on the front of the apparatus. Carbon dioxide was also arranged to flow through the nitrous oxide flowmeter when required. The mixed gases could be passed through chloroform in a 4 oz (100ml) glass bottle (which stood on a square of asbestos to prevent the transfer of

warmth from the hot water canister below: a nice touch and thoughtful, perhaps owing something to a mischievous hint by Charles King himself). The vapours passed through a coil in the hot water bath, thence to a cavity in the wall of the canister before delivery to the patient. The upper reservoir held 'one pound of ether' and a drip fed liquid ether into the cavity mentioned, where it was vaporized by the gas mixture. Neat touches were provided by the 'angled filler for the chloroform bottle which automatically closes the bottle when swung back into place' and by a tap in one of the hollow supports for the ether chamber which 'allowed the pressure in the chamber to be conducted above the surface of the ether in the reservoir so that the gravity feed is effective at all pressures.' A manometer and pressure valve were also fitted.

This apparatus was an ingenious attempt to satisfy a multiplicity of needs within a compact and portable design. Lewis's early death by suicide undoubtedly cut off a practical anaesthetist who would have made further contributions to the specialty.

AI AUSTRALIAN ARMY ENDO-TRACHEAL ETHER APPARATUS, 1939.

This apparatus owes its origin to Dr Geoffrey Kaye, of Melbourne, doyen of Australian anaesthetists and an enthusiastic designer of anaesthetic machinery (Fig. 4.22). The Geoffrey Kaye Museum, now displayed at the Royal Australasian College of Surgeons, is a great collection of anaesthetic apparatus, largely amassed and set out in the first place by Dr Kaye, to whom the author is indebted for his personal friendship and advice.†

---

* Lewis gives 9 in $\times$ $6\frac{1}{2}$ in $\times$ 11 in (23cm $\times$ 16.5cm $\times$ 28cm).

† The present curator of the Geoffrey Kaye Museum is Dr H.Peter Penn, to whom I am also most grateful. K.B.T.

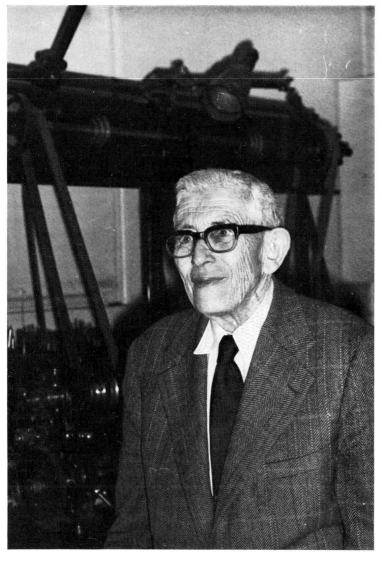

FIG. 4.22. DR GEOFFREY KAYE, MELBOURNE 1975, in his workshop. Founder of the Museum of Anaesthetic Apparatus which now bears his name.

Geoffrey Kaye described this apparatus in the *Australian Army Manual of Anaesthetics*[33] which he wrote while in the Western Desert in 1941. This was a time when relatively untrained and in-experienced anaesthetists were working in forward areas, and simple apparatus with careful descriptions were supplied by the Australian Army, Captain Kaye being the source of their advice.

Writing to the present author in answer to a query Dr Kaye gave an interesting and historical account of the production both of the book and of the apparatus under the difficulties of war.

'The *Army Manual*' he wrote 'was written in Egypt at the end of '41. . . . Although the writer, I was only issued with a single copy and that is the one which is now . . . or ought to be, now . . . in the R.S.M. It wasn't a good manual, but it served its purpose of the time.' Dr Kaye's copy is indeed in the Library of the Royal Society of Medicine.

Of the present apparatus, Dr Kaye wrote 'Australian Army Ether Apparatus. This very simple ether vaporiser was designed (by G. Kaye) for the Australian Army in 1938, and accepted in 1939, just in time for the outbreak of war. It was envisaged that the Australian expeditionary force would operate in the Middle East; that it would depend upon the supplies of gases made in—and shipped from—Australia; that gases might thus be in short supply in the Middle East; and that much 'maintenance' surgery might be done under ether, leaving the gas supply for the battle-casualties. On those terms, the ether vaporizer did quite useful work and ensured that gas-anaesthesia was always available for the sicker patients.

The intention was to produce an apparatus as simple, as rugged and as cheaply as possible. The large diameter and internal baffles provided quite good vaporization of the ether. The enveloping tank served as a 'heat-exchanger', being filled with water at room temperature. The air supply came, in forward units, from a glass-blower's foot bellows: in Hospital units, a rheostat and electric blower (from a field generator) were supplied. The accessories included a reservoir-bag, an expiratory valve (of a bore then deemed adequate, but unduly small by the standards of the 1950's) a set of Magill's elbow tubes, and a laryngoscope.* Magill type endotracheal tubes were made at no. 2 Australian General Hospital, Al-Qantara, from such rubber tubing as was procurable in Cairo. In Field Ambulances, how-ever, even the simple ether vaporizer would have formed an undue burden, so resort was made to a modified form of Flagg's can†. . . . Such cans were made-up in some number at Al Qantara from Army ration cream-tins, and served a useful purpose in forward areas, e.g. in the Tobruk perimeter.

The Army's ether-vaporizer was produced initially, if memory serves, by Messrs Ramsay (Surgical) Ltd. of Melbourne. Later, contracts were placed with divers other firms: the whole apparatus was so simple, even so primitive, that 'anyone' was com-petent to make it.

The example which you hold was probably one donated by the Minister for the Army in 1946, and distributed to what is now the museum of the Faculty of Anaesthetists in Melbourne, to various collections in the U.K. and the U.S.A., and probably

* A laryngoscope of the same pattern is in the Collection (Aust.[3]

† See King Collection No. Aust. 2. p. 49.

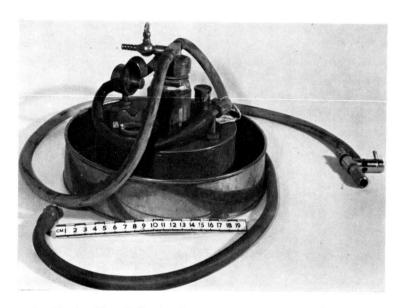

to the Charles King Collection.'*

The apparatus (Figs. 4.23, 4.24) is described in Dr Kaye's *Army Manual*, from which the following notes are taken:

'Air is caused to pass above the surface of ether in a large metal tank eight inches (20 cm) in diameter. A control tap of the circumferential-way type regulates the final strength of the ether vapour by controlling the extent to which the air is admitted to the ether tank. The two streams of air, that traversing the ether tank and that byepassed from it, unite at a common lead and are conducted to a trap bottle. The latter is a safeguard against the entry of liquid ether into the delivery tube, as might occur were the tank overfilled or grossly tilted. It consists of a two-ounce

ointment pot, screwed into a metal cap having inlet and outlet vents. A byepass tap in the cap allows of the addition of oxygen or carbon dioxide. The ether tank possesses a filter cap and a blow-off valve, consisting of a fibre disk on a metal seating with vents opening to the external air above the disc. A threaded cap causes a coil spring to impinge upon the disc . . . the spring will yield under pressures in excess of 40 mm Hg. Escape at lower pressures is arranged by unscrewing the cap the lower edge of which should register against a scale engraved on the barrel of the valve. In the first samples of the apparatus to be accepted by the Army, inspection failed to detect the fact that this calibration had been omitted;† the anaesthetist can however, readily perform it for himself by the aid of a sphygmomano-

* Personal communication from Dr Geoffrey Kaye, Melbourne, 10 April 1969.

† It had been omitted on the Charles King Collection example.

FIG. 4.24. THE AUSTRALIAN
APPARATUS.
Diagram from Kaye, Orton,
Renton. (1946) *Anaesthetic Methods.*
Melbourne: Ramsay. Fig. 57.
(From a copy in the author's
possession).

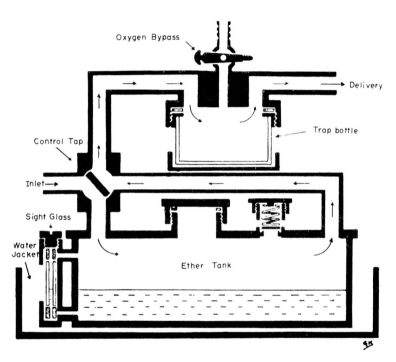

meter and a dental drill.

The tank bears a sight-glass . . . (and) rests in a retaining ring . . . surrounded by a water jacket which will not ordinarily need to be used in the climate of the Middle East. *Ether Concentration,* . . . Thanks to the wide diameter of the tank, the concentration of ether will be found adequate . . . even for anaesthesia for tonsillectomy by insufflation . . . through a Boyle–Davis gag, than which there is no more stringent test of an ether vapour apparatus.

Endopharyngeal administration. For endopharyngeal anaesthesia, the delivery tube may be passed below an ether mask, or connected to a pharyngeal airway, naso-pharyngeal catheter, Boyle–Davis gag or other device.

Endotracheal administration. The Army presupposes the use of endotracheal inhalational anaesthesia by a modification of the Magill technique. To this end, the apparatus is equipped with Magill rubber catheters,* an exhalation valve and a rubber bag (see Fig. 4.25). Endotracheal insufflation anaesthesia through a narrow-bore, gum elastic catheter may, however, be practised if desired. . . .'[33]

* i.e. wide-bore Magill endotracheal tubes.

FIG. 4.25. DIAGRAM OF THE
APPARATUS AS SET UP,
a reservoir bag being included.
From Kaye, Orton, Renton., (1946)
ibid. Fig. 56.

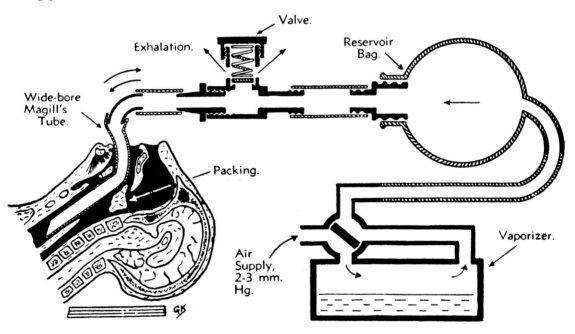

This extract is quoted at some length to show the detail of description required for anaesthetists working in the field in 1941. Other points which may be noticed are that no baffles were thought necessary in the ether tank, and that the diameter of the metal and rubber tubes was one-quarter inch (0.6cm) Noteworthy also is that it was thought necessary to mention insufflation anaesthesia through a narrow-bore catheter, though it is obvious that this practice was not recommended.

As a practical design for use under service conditions, the Australian Army Ether apparatus of Dr Kaye may be compared with its exact contemporary and counterpart, the Oxford Vaporizer, designed in 1941 by Professor Macintosh and Dr Epstein with the aid of Morris Motors. (see p. 9). The British service anaesthetist possibly failed fully to appreciate his good fortune.

Without at all decrying Dr Kaye's design, ruggedly made as it was for cheap and easy production, the refinements inherent in the Oxford design may be compared with the Australian pattern, which lacked a wide-bore system and an integral reservoir bag, and required an external source of pressure. Both owed something of their origin to Flagg's can, (p. 49) and to the wartime need for a simple piece of apparatus without nitrous oxide or oxygen cylinders. Macintosh's apparatus, like that of Flagg, depended on the 'draw-over' principle.

REFERENCES

1 THOMAS K.B. (1970) The A.Charles King Collection of early anesthetic apparatus. *Anaesthesia*. **25**. 556 (item no. 23).

2 POWER D'ARCY (1953) *Lives of the Fellows of the Royal College of Surgeons of England*. London. published by the College. p. 448.

3 Obituary notices: (1944) Sir Robert Kelly. *Brit. med. J*. **ii**. 738. *Lancet* **ii**. 740.

4 MELTZER S.J. & AUER J. (1909) Continuous Respiration without voluntary Movements. *J. Exper. Med*. **11**. 622–625.

5 MELTZER & AUER (1909) *ibid*. p. 624.

6 KELLY R.E. (1911) Intratracheal Anaesthesia. *Brit. J. Surg*. **1**. 90–95.

7 ELSBERG C.A. (1911) Anaesthesia by the Intratracheal Insufflation of Air and Ether. *Annals of Surgery*. **53**. 161.

8 Obituary notices: (1968) Sir Francis Shipway. *Brit. med. J*. **iv**. 649. 780. *Anaesthesia* 1969 **24**. 296.

9 SHIPWAY F.E. (1916) The advantages of warm anaesthetic vapours and an apparatus for their administration. *Lancet*. **i**. 70.

10 PEMBREY M.S. & SHIPWAY F.E. (1916) The Influence of Anaesthetics on the Body Temperature. *Proc. Roy. Soc. Med*. **9** (*Anaesth. Sect.*) p. 3.

11 GWATHMEY J.T. (1912) The Value of Warmed Anaesthetics. *New York Med. J*. **95**. 1130.

12 SEELIG M.G. (1911) The Fallacy of Warmed Ether Vapour. *Interstate med. J*. **18**. 927.

13 TETER G. (1912) Limitations of Nitrous Oxide with Oxygen as a general anaesthetic. *J. Amer. Med. Ass*. **59**. 1849.

14 ROWBOTHAM E.S. & MAGILL I. (1921) Anaesthetics in the Plastic Surgery of the Face and Jaws. *Proc. Roy. Soc. Med*. **14**. pt. I. (*sect. anaesth.*) p. 17.

15 ROWBOTHAM E.S. & MAGILL I.W. (1921). *ibid*.

16 ROWBOTHAM E.S. (1920) Intratracheal anaesthesia through the nose. *Brit. med. J*. **ii**. 590.

17 MAGILL I.M. (1927a) in discussion. Anaesthesia for Dental Surgery. *Proc. Roy. Soc. Med*. **20**. 1301.

18 MAGILL I.W. (1930) Discussion on Anaesthesia in Thoracic Surgery. *Proc. Roy. Soc. Med*. **23**. 779.

19 FEATHERSTONE H.W. (1931) A visit to Canada. . . . *Proc. Roy. Soc. Med*. **24**. 105.

20 ROWBOTHAM E.S. (1926) Intracheal Anaesthesia. *Lancet*. **ii**. 583.

21 ROWBOTHAM E.S. & MAGILL I.W. (1921) *op. cit.*

22 MAGILL I.W. (1921) A Portable Apparatus for Tracheal Insufflation Anaesthesia. *Lancet*. **i**. 918.

23 MAGILL I.W. (1927b) Improved anaesthetic apparatus. *Lancet*. **ii**. 396.

24 MAGILL I.W. (1921) *op. cit.*

25 MAGILL I.W. (1923) An Apparatus for the Administration of Nitrous Oxide, Oxygen and Ether. *Lancet*. **ii**. 228.

26 Personal communication. The late Dr Harold Avery, physician to the Italian Hospital.

27 Obituary notices: (1932) H.R.Phillips. *Lancet*. **i**. 1388. *Brit. med. J*. **i**. 1194.

28 PHILLIPS H.R. (1916a) Anaesthesia for Enucleation of Tonsils. *Lancet*. **i**. 838.

29 PHILLIPS H.R. (1916b) Anaesthesia for Two Cases of Patent Ductus. *Lancet*. **i**. 1124.

30 PHILLIPS H.R. (1918) Apparatus for Administering oxygen with ether and chloroform. *Proc. Roy. Soc. Med*. **11**. (*Anaesth. Sect.* p. 13).

31 Obituary notice: (1938) Ivor Nicholas Lewis. *St. George's Hospital Gazette*. p. 169.

32 LEWIS I. (1931) Apparatus for Anaesthesia. *Lancet*. **ii**. 1304.

33 KAYE G. (1942) *Manual of Army Anaesthetic Apparatus*. Australian Military Forces. Melbourne.

Section V
Mixed Vapours

ILLUSTRATIONS

INTRODUCTION: *ALCOHOL AS A VEHICLE*

With the realization by 1848 of the dangers of the newly introduced chloroform, differing reactions took place in different places. In America there was an almost complete return to the use of ether, if indeed that drug had ever been forsaken. It was natural that chloroform should be banned at the Massachusetts General Hospital, the birthplace of ether anaesthesia, and the rest of North America followed. In France too, chloroform deaths in Lyons and other towns produced a renunciation of its use, as also in most of Italy[1].

In England, there was a move to persevere with the use of chloroform. Even John Snow continued to use the drug on account of its convenience, though admitting its dangers, and the relative safety of ether; according to his biographer, Benjamin Ward Richardson, Snow said—'I use chloroform for the same reason that you use phosphorus matches instead of the tinder box. An occasional risk never stands in the way of ready applicability'[2]. This attitude was adopted by many English anaesthetists and for the rest of the century, apparatus for use with chloroform was studied and developed in England.

Others, however, suggested that mixtures of ether and chloroform might be of value, each drug counteracting the disadvantages of the other. Charles Kidd of London reported the use of the well-known Vienna mixture in 1859, saying that it was composed of one part of chloroform to six or eight of ether[3].

As early as 1848, John Gabb of Bewdley suggested that it 'might be desirable to add a little of the stimulating effect of the ether to the directly sedative influence of the chloroform. Could not this be done'

he asked 'by mixing the two agents . . . about one part of ether to two parts of chloroform'[4].

Mr Vaughan Jones of Westminster answered Gabb by suggesting that this 'would not be found practicable on account of the difference in specific gravity of the two agents: so that unless an ether-and-chloroform apparatus could be invented, the advantages expected by Mr Gabb . . . cannot possibly be arrived at'[5].

This was but a partial answer: the real cause of the problems of mixtures was given by Snow. In his great book posthumously published, which covers all the then known aspects of chloroform anaesthesia, is his opinion on *the Combination of Chloroform and Ether*: 'the result of mixtures', said Snow in his best incisive manner, is 'a combination of the undesirable qualities of both agents, without any compensating advantage. Ether is about six times as volatile as chloroform . . . and when the two liquids are mixed, although they then evaporate together, the ether is converted into vapour much more rapidly . . . the consequence is that at the commencement of an inhalation the vapour inspired is chiefly ether, and towards the end nearly all chloroform: the patient experiencing the stronger pungency of ether when it is most objectionable, and inhaling the more powerful vapour at the conclusion when there is most need to proceed cautiously'[6]. Snow could be both pungent and powerful.

In spite of this caveat, which indeed had become common knowledge, the idea of mixed anaesthetics flourished.

Among those advocating their use was George Harley, 1829–96, distinguished Harley Street physician and investigator of anaesthetic and other drugs, including curare. About 1860, Harley suggested the use of the mixture which became famous as the 'A.C.E.' mixture, these being the initial letters of its constituents, alcohol, one part: chloroform, 2 parts: ether, 3 parts: this mixture continued in use until well into the present century.

By 1864, chloroform fatalities had reached such a level that the first of a long series of investigations was set up. Under the chairmanship of the surgeon, George Curling, the Royal Medical and Chirurgical Society (which became the Royal Society of Medicine in 1905) set up its Chloroform Committee. Among its members were George Harley, Francis Sibson, Benjamin Ward Richardson and Charles Kidd, all of whom were practising anaesthetists, and all of whom had contributed scientific work to the specialty. In addition, Joseph Clover, 'attended at their request all the meetings for experiments, administered the chloroform and contrived, from time to time, with remarkable ingenuity, special apparatus for carrying them out,' to quote from the lengthy report which appeared in the *Medico-Chirurgical Transactions*[7, 8].

From its experimental work on dogs, the Committee reached conclusions regarding the relative safety of chloroform and ether almost identical with those which John Snow had already propounded[9].

Finally, the Committee recommended the use of mixtures, having found 'alarming symptoms' (in dogs), from the use of chloroform, and concurring 'in the general opinion which in this country has led to the disuse of ether as an inconvenient anaesthetic'[7].

Three mixtures were investigated. Mixture A, which was George Harley's A.C.E. prescription: mixture B, consisting of chloroform/ether in 1:4 proportions: mixture C, chloroform/ether, 1:2.

Mixture B was found to be 'very similar in its physiological effects to simple ether . . . the chief objection being the slowness of its operation.' Mixtures A and C were found to be very similar to each other, their actions being 'intermediate between that of chloroform and ether . . . insensibility might be induced with sufficient rapidity; in from four to eight minutes in animals and in from ten to fifteen minutes in man.' The report commented upon the relative rates of evaporation, but laid no particular stress upon this important finding.

The results of the Committee's workings were twofold. Firstly, most physicians practising anaesthesia continued to use chloroform; but, as Duncum points out, there began a weakening of the position of the drug. The search for other anaesthetics was abandoned: the return to ether began.

Secondly, some anaesthetists used both drugs, either in sequence or as actual mixtures. Robert Ellis produced the first mixture apparatus; this will be described. Others tried the A.C.E. mixture of Harley, which continued long in use. A survey of some of the anaesthetic textbooks of the late nineteenth century is not without interest.

Sansom, 1865[10], described the recommendations of the 1864 Committee, suggesting that from his own experiments 'the alcohol (in the A.C.E. mixture) had the greatest effect in sustaining the heart's action during the influence of chloroform.' Thus the old 'stimulation' idea was still alive.

Underwood, 1885[11], of the Dental Hospital, London, wrote of 'the stimulating properties of the ether being supposed to counteract the depressant effect of the chloroform.' Cautiously he stated that experimental work on these matters should be left to the experts, and, with considerable forbearance, added 'as this book is not addressed to privileged experts, I shall not uselessly occupy the reader's time by discussing the matter further.'

Dudley Buxton, 1888[12], from University College Hospital, London, devoted a whole chapter to mixtures; he discussed A.C.E., the Vienna mixture,

Linhart's (alcohol/chloroform 1:4) and Billroth's (chloroform/ether/alcohol, 3:1:1): and described Ellis's apparatus (p. 216) as 'too complicated for practical purposes: the method has never received much favour.' Buxton favoured Harley's A.C.E. mixture, which 'may be given in a Clover's ether-inhaler, a cone, or even by the open method,' mentioning also that deaths have occurred during the use of the A.C.E. mixture. He did however, quote the disadvantage of unequal evaporation. Billroth's mixture was used with a Junker's inhaler (p. 73); special care was needed with so strong a chloroform mixture. Of interest, too are Buxton's comments on using chloroform and ether with alkaloids, etc.; for example, the use of morphine before both chloroform and ether is discussed. He described its satisfactory use with chloroform, mentioning the dangers of asphyxia and inhalation of blood in pharyngeal haemorrhage. He recommended the use of atropine to paralyze the vagus which he says 'might be a valuable antidote to chloroform, by preventing reflex inhibition of the heart.' This was E.A.Schafer's recommendation of 1880[13], and it is interesting to note that modern practice has returned full circle to the use of atropine for this purpose, after a long interval when its use was mainly for its antisialogogue action. Buxton also mentioned chloroform and chloral—'I cannot think the advantages . . . in any way counterbalance the dangers . . .', and ether with chloral—'a death has occurred.' He finished his chapter on mixtures with a mention of nitrous oxide and ether, 'the best method of producing general anaesthesia'; thus indicating that consideration of mixtures in general may have had some bearing on the thoughts of those such as Clover, who advocated nitrous oxide sequences. (p. 121).

Others who discussed mixtures included Probyn-Williams, Instructor in Anaesthetics at the London Hospital, (p. 28) who gave a useful account in 1909 in which he wrote 'the use of the alcohol in the mixture has given rise to much discussion. It acts as a diluent of the chloroform and is said to lead to a more intimate connection between the chloroform and ether, and to make the mixture more stable than one of ether and chloroform alone.'

'Some administrators consider that it is unsatisfactory to work with two drugs, without knowing the exact proportion of each one that is being administered: for the ether evaporates more quickly than the chloroform, while the alcohol remains till the last. This is undoubtedly to a great extent true, though the alcohol prevents the ether from evaporating as fast as it would if it were only mixed with chloroform.'

'The character of the anaesthesia it produces lies midway between those procured by means of its two principal constituents . . . a quiet sleep is obtained resembling that of chloroform, while circulatory depression is less marked: in fact the pulse generally improves soon after the substitution of this mixture for chloroform. It may be given alone throughout the operation, or simply as a pleasant start for the administration of ether: and it is also most useful when a change is required on account of the amount of secretion produced by the latter drug'[14]. The mixture was given either on an open mask such as Skinner's (King Collection No. 50, Fig. 7.3) or with the cone-type semi-open Rendle or Silk mask (King Collection No. 64, p. 43).

Such were the thoughts upon mixtures in 1909 of an experienced practitioner and teacher of anaesthetics. Bellamy Gardner, of Charing Cross Hospital, 1916, voiced exactly the same opinions[15], as did Blomfield, of St George's Hospital in 1917[16].

Hadfield, of St Bartholomew's Hospital, in 1923

described the use of a modified Rendle's mask, and then condemned it for the possibility of sudden overdosage if a deep inspiration is taken after a period of breath holding[17].

As late as 1944, the sixth edition of the textbook of Minnitt and Gillies[18] stated that a servicable mixture was that known as C_2E_3, and made the sage and belated observation that 'a heart poisoned by excess of chloroform does not respond to ether stimulation.' These authors suggested Hewitt's sequence of *Chloroform/ether to closed-ether* as a means of dealing with alcoholic men. The present writer recalls that C_2E_3 was used at Hewitt's old hospital, Charing Cross, in the late 1930's. Looking back with some awe at such temerity, one is tempted to follow Minnitt and Gillies with a quotation from the late Professor Leonard Hill:

'Chloroform is a drug used by the young anaesthetist with the utmost hardihood, and until he has had the misfortune to meet with a death by it, he derides the danger of the drug, and asserts that its safety merely depends on the care and skill of the administrator. After losing his patient, he falls to discanting on the unavoidable dangers of the drug, dangers which he is now the first to maintain cannot be met by any degree of skill in administration.'

This history of mixtures of liquid anaesthetics cannot be concluded without brief reference to the peculiar resurrection, some sixteen years ago, of a precisely similar mixture, the azeotropic mixture of ether with halothane. The original paper appears to have been that of Hudon and Jacques, presented at the Annual Meeting of the Canadian Anaesthetists Society, Montebello, Quebec, 20 June 1958[19]. Dobkin and his colleagues followed with a definitive clinical study[20], but Lee and Atkinson now say 'the consensus of opinion is that the azeotrope has little or no superiority over halothane alone'[21], a statement which might have produced a wry and understanding smile from John Snow.

CKC 5: ELLIS ALCOHOL-ETHER-CHLOROFORM APPARATUS 1866

Robert Ellis, L.S.A., 1844, described himself in his book and papers as Obstetric Surgeon to the Chelsea, Brompton and Belgrave Dispensaries, and he practised from Sloane Street, Chelsea. No obituary notices have been found, but his name does not appear in the *Medical Directory* after 1885. In 1866 he published a small book entitled *On the Safe Abolition of Pain in Labour*[22] (Fig. 5.1) in which he described a piece of apparatus for anaesthesia in midwifery by the use of the mixed effects of chloroform, ether and alcohol (Fig. 5.2). In the same year Ellis also published several papers in the *Lancet*[23, 24, 25], in which the virtues of 'mixed vapours' were extolled, and in which the apparatus in various forms was described. (Figs. 5.3, 5.4, 5.5). A few quotations from these papers show Ellis's viewpoint:

'I think probably few are in the habit of exhibiting chloroform without a sense of doubt as to the manner in which it will take effect. . . . The risk is small: . . . Death by spasm and death by paralysis of the heart may probably be set down as the principal causes of a fatal issue arising out of the use of undiluted chloroform. . . . Reflecting on the commoner causes of fatal chloroform accidents, the conviction is impressed on me that we commence our anaesthetic induction with the wrong agency. Chloroform, however diluted, is unsuitable for the early stages of inhalation and it is in these especially, as e.g. in the recent fatal accident at St Mary's—that fatal results have been most frequent'[23]. After

SAFE ABOLITION OF PAIN

IN

LABOUR AND SURGICAL OPERATIONS,

BY

ANÆSTHESIA WITH MIXED VAPOURS.

BY

ROBERT ELLIS,

SURGEON-ACCOUCHEUR TO THE CHELSEA, BROMPTON, AND BELGRAVE DISPENSARY;
AUTHOR OF "DISEASE IN CHILDHOOD," ETC.

LONDON:
ROBERT HARDWICKE, 192 PICCADILLY.

1866.

FIG. 5.1. TITLE PAGE OF ROBERT ELLIS'S BOOK, 1866.
From a copy in the author's possession.

FIG. 5.2. ELLIS ALCOHOL-ETHER-
CHLOROFORM APPARATUS, 1866.
Note the three fillers and compare
Fig. 5.4. At the base of the wide-
bore breathing tube is an
occluding air hole.
CKC 5

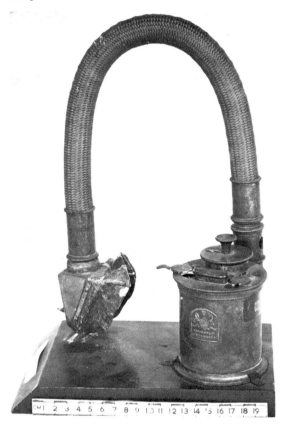

describing his method of mixing vapours in this apparatus, Ellis went on. . . . 'For prolonged anaesthesia, as in obstetric practice, I think this apparatus admirably adapted.

After a partial anaesthetic effect is produced by the mixed vapours it is then easy to turn on a little more chloroform with each wave of uterine effort and to turn it off to the safer vapour again as the 'pain' subsides. By this means we obtain all the advantages claimed by the Chloroform Committee

for their anaesthetic mixtures, with the additional one of having the potent agent most completely under our control'[23].

Ellis therefore propounded the idea that, as chloroform was a depressant, the Chloroform Committee* having said so, it was more appropriate to initiate the anaesthetic with 'stimulating' drugs, e.g. alcohol and ether. It has to be remembered, moreover, that in using the term 'anaesthesia', Ellis, at least in his obstetric practice, was referring to a state more resembling that which we should now term 'analgesia'.

Ellis took great trouble to point out that the volatilization of mixed anaesthetic fluids was 'independent each of the other, and in extremely differing quantities,' adding 'for a considerable time past I have endeavoured to impress this fact on the notice of my professional brethren and to show that there is a more excellent anaesthetic method by which perfect security can be obtained, and definite and known quantities of the anaesthetic agents administered. This is the method of separate evaporation of these fluids and administration of the mixed vapours'[26].

How did Ellis arrange this? His apparatus is neat and well thought out, though he says he made his own original model from a few bits of brass tubing. The first design (Fig. 5.3) consisted of an upper wide cylinder, about 5cm in diameter with a smaller tube fitted to its base. The whole was divided by a metal partition, on one side of which chloroform was placed, and on the other alcohol and ether. (Ellis makes a great point of the need for purity of the liquids). The lower part of the smaller tube has an elliptical opening which communicates with the long

---

* Committee on Chloroform of the Royal Medical and Chirurgical Society, 1864. (See introduction to this Section, p. 212).

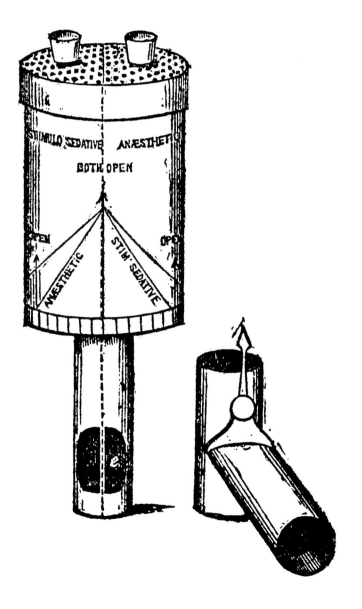

FIG. 5.3. EARLY FORM OF ELLIS
VAPORIZER.
From Ellis, R. (1866)
Anaesthesia by Mixed Vapours.
Lancet, **i**, 145.

arm of a T-tube, on which an indicator shows the positions of the openings, the 'scale having been adjusted by experiment'[23].

The development of this apparatus produced a new idea, that of using capillary attraction, and it is this later model which is represented in the King Collection (No. 5, Fig. 5.2).

Fig. 5.4 shows a top view of the inhaler, the cover and control drum being removed. The latter rotates in the tube *a* to open or close the quarter circle ports. These in turn communicate with the chloroform sector *c* and with the ether sector *d*. In each of these a small glass test tube contains the anaesthetic liquid, which vaporizes from the wicks shown in the figures. Alcohol is vaporized from a cage covered with thin linen gauze, and this compartment is in communication with the ether chamber, though not with the chloroform. A wide-bore exit tube with perforated ring for admission of air; an eighteen inch wide-bore non-kinking tube of fabric covered rubber with a special internal wire, and brass sockets: and a Snow type face piece of brass and leather, with inspiratory and expiratory valves, complete the apparatus. The whole is beautifully made. Air is drawn through the apparatus by two holes with covers acting also as chloroform and ether fillers, each $\frac{1}{2}$ in (1.3cm) in diameter and by an oblong hole $1\frac{1}{8}$ in $\times$ 3 in (2.9cm $\times$ 1cm). The inhaling areas are thus insufficient for unembarrassed respiration even when all three are open. The oblong alcohol slot is never closed, and one or other of the others may be opened, according to the requirements of adding ether or chloroform or both. In practice the efficiency is not high since a good deal of leakage of air occurs.

Ellis made much of the method of capillary attraction. At a meeting of the Obstetric Society of London he 'drew attention to two very important

features . . . the first (being) the method of only liberating a certain number of minims per minute of chloroform or ether. This was effected by an adaptation of the self-acting law of capillary attraction: and the other was the powerful evaporating surface of a frilled description, by which the inspired air can be saturated with the powerfully stimulant vapour of alcohol. . . . So great was this economy of use that in anaesthesia in such an operation as ovariotomy, extending over half an hour, scarcely two drachms (6ml) of chloroform were used . . . or only three quarters per cent of chloroform in the inspired air'[27].

The apparatus is shown in an elegant little engraving, in use during labour (Fig. 5.6) and Ellis made the point that it may be left in the charge of the midwife. (Compare the story of 1933, p. 234).

In another version of the apparatus, described as *Mr Robt. Ellis's Obstetric Inhaler*, (Fig. 5.5), the chloroform drips from a wick in the bottle placed on top of the ether/alcohol chamber, and Ellis provided an almost ecstatic description . . . 'the beautiful regularity with which this most simple instrument performs its required office must be seen to be appreciated' and 'so soon as these facts shall become known and mixed anaesthetics more generally used. . . . I believe the napkin and tumbler system of giving chloroform, especially in midwifery, will drop out of knowledge and practice'[28].

It is perhaps unfortunate that Ellis's enthusiasm was not communicated to the rest of the profession; his apparatus seems not to have been commented upon by others. After 1866, he appears to have taken no further interest in anaesthesia, perhaps in accordance with a remark in one of his papers: 'Not having a desire to win a reputation for giving anaesthetics only, I am unable to devote much time to making this method known'[29].

FIG. 5.4. Top view of Ellis
vaporizer to show rotating control,
a, h, g; ether and chloroform wicks
in small test tubes, c, d: and
alcohol wick, e.
From Ellis, R., (1866) *On the Safe
Abolition of Pain in Labour*.
London: Hardwicke, p. 76

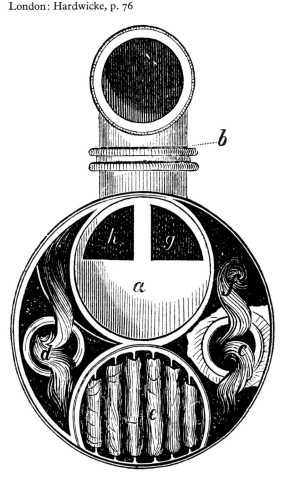

CKC 48: BRAUN ETHER-CHLOROFORM VAPORIZER 1901

This vaporizer (Fig. 5.7) was labelled 'Röth-Dräger, 1903' by Charles King and his attribution was copied into the *Inventory* of 1970. Gwathmey, (1905)[30], Kocher, (1911)[31], and Kirschner, (1931)3[2], each show and describe apparatus identical with the present, ascribing it to H.Braun of Leipsig, and this can be confirmed from his own description, given below. Kocher said that Braun used chloroform for induction and maintained anaesthesia with ether—'once anaesthesia is obtained the majority of patients can be kept under its influence by giving small but repeated administrations of ether.'

The apparatus is a modification of Junker's (see CKC 17, 63, A17, p. 73) in which a current of air is used to carry ether or chloroform or both, the flow being separately controlled. (Figs. 5.8, 5.9). Two bottles of brown glass, one calibrated to 50cu cm the other to 150cu cm, are mounted side by side in an open wire cage; to the metal collars of their mouths is clamped a metal casting from the lower outer ends of which a tube passes into each bottle. The casting is bored out to allow for taps to control the flow to the bottles, and for inlet and outlet tubes (Fig. 5.8). The inlet tube connects to a hand bellows, as in Junker's apparatus, and the outlet tube to a valveless metal mask.

H.Braun of Göttingen described this apparatus in 1901, a report subsequently appearing in the *British Medical Journal*: 'he uses a minimum quantity of chloroform vapour in normal cases, merely using a full mixture until a marked tolerance is shown: after this the chloroform tap may be turned off'[33]. Braun reported anaesthetizing 250 patients using an average of 54cu cm ether and 12cu cm chloroform. There were no disagreeable or dangerous symptoms

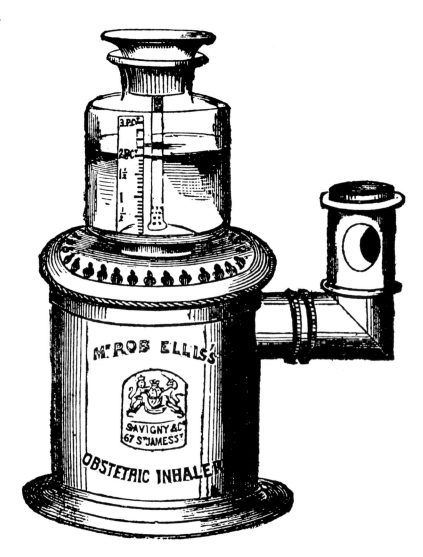

FIG. 5.5. ELLIS DRIP-
CHLOROFORM INHALER:
ether and alcohol in lower chamber.
Ellis, R. (1866) Compound
Anaesthetics in Midwifery. *Lancet*
i, 708

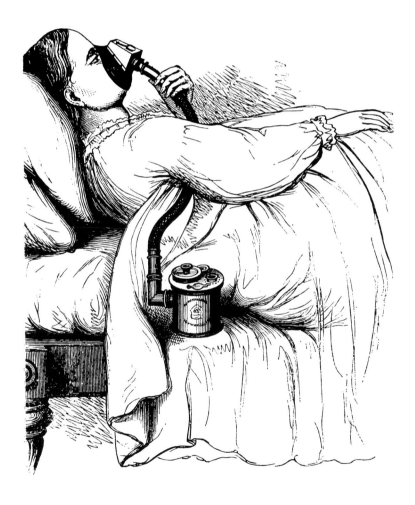

FIG. 5.6. ELLIS VAPORIZER IN
USE, 1866
From *The Safe Abolition of Pain in
Labour*, 1866, p. 79

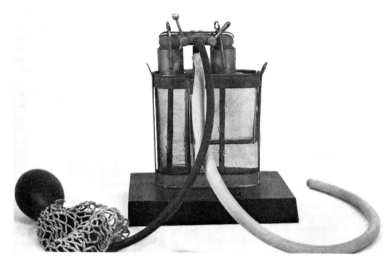

FIG. 5.7. BRAUN ETHER-CHLOROFORM VAPORIZER, 1901. Two springs hold down the cap, from which dip-tubes pass to the chloroform (left) and ether (right) bottles, each having a control lever. Air from a pressure source (left hand tube) (see Figs. 5.8., 5.9.,) carries the mixed vapours through the narrow-bore tube (right) to the face mask.
CKC 48 (labelled Röth-Drager).

even though 'the anaesthetists were only partly experienced.'

This was a piece of apparatus which had a vogue. Gwathmey had used it over 200 times (with a Hewitt face mask) 'and on each occasion with an increased degree of satisfaction to myself'[30]. He added 'Dr Braun's idea is to give a continual anaesthesia by means of a highly attenuated ether vapour, to which, from time to time, chloroform is added. . . . The Braun apparatus is simple and easy to operate and has decided advantages over the Harcourt Inhaler (CKC 20, page 86). But the principal and greatest objection to these, and to all other inhalers up to this time, is that the air or oxygen cannot be increased or decreased, without at the same time increasing or decreasing the anaesthetic vapour.' From this point Gwathmey went on to produce his own mixed vapour inhaler, which preceded his later nitrous oxide/oxygen machine of 1912 (CKC 24, p. 141).

It seems that Braun's apparatus was little used in

England, and the provenance of the present specimen is unknown. Nor is it known why Charles King should have called it *Röth-Dräger*. Röth of Lübeck had introduced a form of 'bubble bottle' in which oxygen was passed through chloroform. This was manufactured by the Lübeck firm of Dräger[34] and was described by Dumont in 1903[35]. However, this apparatus bears no resemblance to the Braun, and though the latter may have been manufactured by Dräger, no connection with Röth has been found.

CKC A16: DE FORD SOMNOFORM(E) INHALER 1908

William Harper De Ford A.M., D.D.S., M.D., was Professor of Oral Pathology and Anaesthetics, Drake University College of Dentistry, Iowa. His published lectures[36] include an enthusiastic description of the use of somnoform with this apparatus.

Somnoform had been introduced in 1901 by Dr

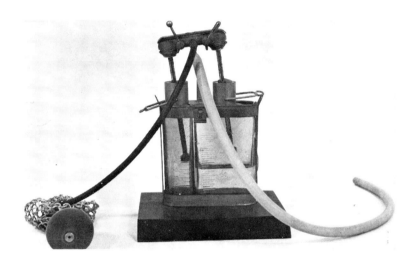

FIG. 5.8. BRAUN ETHER-CHLOROFORM VAPORIZER, 1901. The top has been lifted to show the dip-tubes, which have only one emitting hole. CKC 48 (labelled Röth-Drager).

Georges Rolland, Director of the Dental School in Bordeaux who had been 'Theoretical and Practical Professor of Anaesthesia' from 1895. A detailed paper[37] was read for him by Mr Field Robinson, L.D.S.I., also of Bordeaux, at the Annual Meeting of the British Dental Association at Shrewsbury, May 1902.

The mixture to which the name *Somnoform(e)* was given is described as being composed of 60 parts of chloride of ethyl, 35 parts of chloride of methyl, and 5 parts of bromide of ethyl (earlier mixtures had contained 12 parts of the latter). 'The research and composition of Somnoforme' it is stated 'are the natural consequence of the didactic functions of Dr Rolland,' whose requirements in an anaesthetic are listed as:

'1. no cumbersome apparatus—something simple
2. instantaneous action
3. rapid elimination, rapid return of consciousness
4. security both in the beginning, during and after effects.'

Field Robinson said 'He resorted to the old method of mixing and thus demanded that each one should give its help to procure the final object. . . . From the diffusibility of chloride of methyl, which evaporates at 23 degrees below zero (and which was the first general anaesthetic he employed for dental purposes) he demanded instantaneous anaesthetical action. From chloride of ethyl, (the base of the anaesthetic), he demanded the prolongation of the transient or fugitive action of the chloride of methyl and finally, from bromide of ethyl, used in feeble proportions of 5 per cent, he demanded the prolongation of the time required for operating by producing an analgesic condition which is a transition between absolute anaesthesia and the return, sometime too rapid, to consciousness and sensibility.'

'Nothing of this seemed to be in contradiction with the indications of general physiology concerning the subjects of respiration, circulation and enervation'[37].

After some rather dubious physico-physiological

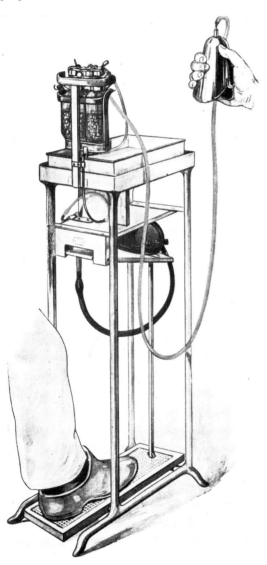

FIG. 5.9. Braun ether-chloroform vaporizer, as used, with foot blower, and valveless metal face mask. From Kirschner, M. (1931) *Operative Surgery*, trans. Ravdin, p. 136

arguments, Field Robinson stated that he had induced anaesthesia (the guinea-pig was Dr Rolland) in 12 seconds. Since the number of patients attending Dr Rolland's clinic each Thursday morning was between 100 and 150, this paper produced a very large number of observations. The vapour was inhaled from a 'cornet, made out of a simple handkerchief, the only apparatus we employ.'

The paper of Field Robinson and Rolland attracted a good deal of attention, and H.E.G.Boyle, then Junior Resident Anaesthetist, read a paper to the Abernethian Society of St Bartholomew's Hospital, on 3 December, 1903[38].

Boyle opined that this anaesthetic would, in a few years 'be more universally adopted by the medical profession than it has been at present.' He employed a celluloid face piece, containing a piece of lint, attached to a rubber bag, and somnoform was used not only alone, but as a precursor to ether or chloroform: this technique had already been described by W.J.McCardie of Birmingham, using an ethyl chloride-ether sequence[39]. It seems curious that none of those who recommended somnoform realized that they obtained their main effects from ethyl chloride. Boyle recorded that 'during the first few breaths patients usually experience a feeling of anguish', which hardly seems to recommend the practice, but an indication of the needs of the time is shown by his statements that 'the average time taken to produce anaesthesia is about forty seconds' and 'the average length of time for working is roughly about ninety to one hundred and twenty seconds, which is longer than is usual with nitrous oxide. . . .' Longer anaesthesia was obtained, up to twenty minutes,' by re-charging and re-applying the face-piece directly signs of returning consciousness appear'[38].

McCardie, who was the ethyl chloride authority,

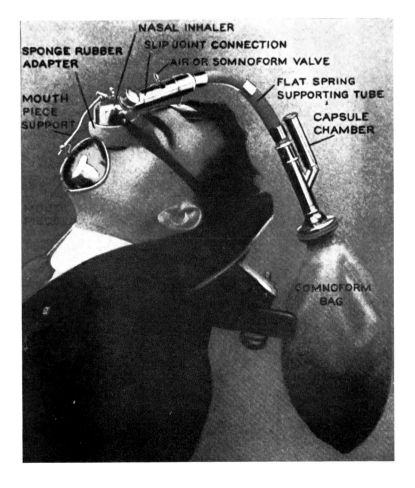

SPONGE RUBBER ADAPTER

MOUTH PIECE SUPPORT

NASAL INHALER

SLIP JOINT CONNECTION

AIR OR SOMNOFORM VALVE

FLAT SPRING SUPPORTING TUBE

CAPSULE CHAMBER

SOMNOFORM BAG

FIG. 5.10. DE FORD SOMNOFORM INHALER IN USE.

A capsule of somnoform is cracked in the capsule chamber and the liquid runs down into the bag, whence its vapour is rebreathed. Air is admitted as required. The mouth cover prevents oral respiration.

From De Ford, W.H. (1912).
Lectures on General Anaesthetics.

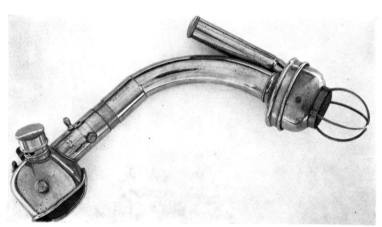

FIG. 5.11. DE FORD SOMNOFORM
INHALER, 1908.
The rebreathing bag is missing.
CKC A16

saw little advantage in somnoform, and believed it to be less safe than pure ethyl chloride[39]. Remarking that there had been seven deaths under ethyl chloride he stated 'there have been a few deaths under somnoform, which was claimed to be an absolutely safe drug . . . but this I take it, is to be considered another anaesthetic.' (i.e. from ethyl chloride).

The present apparatus (Figs. 5.10, 5.11) was first produced in 1908 and bears the patent number 1755, July 7, 1908, Stratford Cookson Co., Philadelphia. A similar specimen in the Geoffrey Kaye Museum. Faculty of Anaesthetists, Melbourne, was manufactured by E.DeTrey and Sons of Philadelphia.*

The apparatus consists of a neat pipe-like tube, 12 in (25cm) in length, curved to fit over the head. A shaped nose-piece is fitted at one end and a one gallon (4.5 litre) rebreathing bag at the distal end. Near this a side tube is attached, in which a capsule of

somnoform is placed. An expiratory valve is fitted to the nose-piece which may also support a mouth occluding cap. Air may be admitted through a small variable orifice of maximum diameter 1cm, through which also incremental doses of somnoform may also be squirted from a spring-cap bottle. The main tube is of wide-bore, 2cm in diameter. The whole is beautifully manufactured, and one suspects that the failure of popularity of somnoform lay in the curious blend involved in that mixture, rather than in this piece of apparatus.

W.H.Archer reported in 1945, that 'this irrational mixture was denied acceptance in 1931 by the (American) Council of Therapeutics'[40].

* Information and photographs kindly supplied by Dr Geoffrey Kaye, and Dr H.P.Penn, Curator, Geoffrey Kaye Museum. Faculty of Anaesthetists, Royal Australian College of Surgeons, Melbourne.

REFERENCES

1 SNOW J. (1858) *On Chloroform and other Anaesthetics.* London: Churchill. p. 23.

2 RICHARDSON B.W. (1858) In Snow, J. *On Chloroform and other Anaesthetics.* London: Churchill, p. xxxv.

3 KIDD C. (1859) *On Aether and Chloroform.* London: Renshaw. 2nd ed. pp. 14. 42.

4 GABB J. (1848) Employment of Ether and Chloroform in Conjunction. *Lancet.* **i.** 521.

5 JONES V. (1848) The Administration of Chloroform and Ether in Conjunction. *Lancet.* **i.** 610.

6 SNOW J. (1858) *op. cit.* p. 369.

7 Report of the Committee appointed by the Royal Medical and Chirurgical Society to inquire into the uses and the Physiological, Therapeutical and Toxical effects of Chloroform (1864). *Med-Chir-Trans.* **47.** 323–442.

8 DUNCUM B. (1947) *Development of Inhalation Anaesthesia.* London: Oxford Univ. Press. p. 253.

9 SNOW J. (1858) *op. cit.* pp. 120. 362 and passim.

10 SANSOM A.E. (1865) *Chloroform, its action and administration.* London: Churchill.

11 UNDERWOOD A.S. (1885) *Notes on Anaesthetics.* London: Ash.

12 BUXTON D.W. (1888) *Anaesthetics, their uses and Administration.* London: Lewis.

13 SCHAFER E.A. (1880) Atropine as a Preventive against the Cardio-Inhibitory effects of chloroform. *Brit. med. J.* **ii.** 620. 761.

14 PROBYN-WILLIAMS R.J. (1909) *Practical Guide to the Administration of Anaesthetics.* London: Longmans, Green. 2nd ed.

15 GARDNER H.B. (1916) *A Manual of Surgical Anaesthesia.* Toronto and London: Macmillan. 2nd ed.

16 BLOMFIELD J. (1917) *Anaesthetics.* London: Baillière, Tindall and Cox. 4th ed.

17 HADFIELD C.F. (1923) *Practical Anaesthetics.* London: Baillière, Tindall and Cox. p. 174.

18 MINNITT R.J. & GILLIES J. (1944) *Textbook of Anaesthetics.* Edinburgh: Livingstone. 6th ed.

19 HUDON F., JACQUES A. (1958) Fluothane-ether mixtures. *Canad. Anaesth. Soc. J.* **5.** 384.

20 DOBKIN A.B., DRUMMOND K., PURKIN N. (1959) Anaesthesia with the Azeotropic Mixture of Halothane and Diethyl Ether. *Brit. J. Anaesth.* **31.** 53.

21 LEE J.A., ATKINSON R.S. (1973) *A Synopsis of Anaesthesia.* Bristol. Wright. 7th ed. p. 214.

22 ELLIS R. (1866a) *On the Safe Abolition of Pain in Labour.* London: Hardwicke.

23 ELLIS R. (1866b) On Anaesthesia by Mixed Vapours. *Lancet.* **i.** 144.

24 ELLIS R. (1866c) Additional note on Anaesthesia by Mixed Vapours. *Lancet.* **i.** 509.

25 ELLIS R. (1866d) Compound Anaesthetics in Midwifery. *Lancet.* **i.** 708.

26 ELLIS R. (1867) On Chloroform and Ether in Mixture. *Med. Times and Gaz.* **i.** 246.

27 ELLIS R. (1866e) Report of meeting in *Lancet.* 1866. **ii.** 151.

28 ELLIS R. (1866d) *op. cit.*

29 ELLIS R. (1866c) *op. cit.*

30 GWATHMEY J.T. (1905) The Vapour Method of Anaesthesia. *Medical Record.* **68.** 609.

31 KOCHER T. (1911) *Textbook of Operative Surgery.* London: Black. 3rd Eng. ed. trans. Stiles and Paul. p. 14–16.

32 KIRSCHNER M. (1931) *Operative Surgery.* trans. Ravdin. Philadelphia and London: Lippincott. p. 136–7.

33 [BRAUN H.[(1901) Ether and Chloroform Anaesthetic Mixture. *Brit. med J.* **i.** *Epitome of current med. lit.* 96.

34 DUNCUM B. (1947) *op. cit.* p. 518.

35 DUMONT F.L. (1903) *Handbuch der allgemeinen und lokalen Anaesthesie.* Berlin. p. 141.

36 DE FORD W.H. (1912) *Lectures on General Anaesthetics in Dentistry, advocating Painless Dental Operations by the Use of Nitrous Oxid, nitrous oxid and Oxygen, Chloroform, Ether, Ethyl Chloride, and Somnoform.* Pittsburg. Lee S.Smith. 2nd ed.

37 ROLLAND G., & ROBINSON F. (1902) Somnoforme, *J. Brit. Dent. Ass.* **23.** 321.

38 BOYLE H.E.G. (1904)
Somnoform Anaesthesia. *St.
Barts. Hosp. J.* **11**. 51–56.
39 McCARDIE W.J. (1905) Ethyl
Chloride as a General
Anaesthetic. *Lancet.* **ii**. 1024.
40 ARCHER W.H. (1945) Historical
Sketch of Anaesthesia. Pt. II.
*Current Researches in Anesthesia
and Analgesia.* **24**. 24.

Section VI
The Analgesia Story

ILLUSTRATIONS

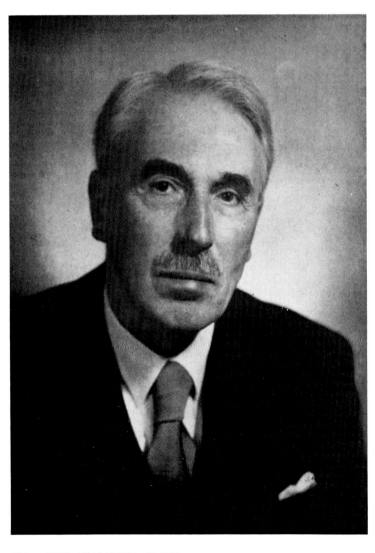

FIG. 6.1. DR ROBERT JAMES
MINNITT 1889–1974.

INTRODUCTION: *LESSENED PAIN IN LYING-IN*

The introduction of chloroform into obstetrics by James Young Simpson in 1847 has been briefly discussed, (p. 59). Within a short time, it was realized by John Snow, Edward Murphy, and others, (p. 65) that the process was one in which full anaesthesia was neither necessary nor desirable. Though Snow understood the successive stages of anaesthesia, with their signs, he was also to write 'when the practice of inhalation in midwifery was first introduced by Dr Simpson, he very naturally adopted the plan which is usually followed in surgical operations, making the patient unconscious at once, and keeping her so to the end of her labour. It was soon found however, by other practitioners that this is not necessary: and indeed it would not be safe in protracted cases. Drs Murphy and Rigby* were, I believe, amongst the first to state, that relief from pain may often be afforded in obstetric cases, without removing the consciousness of the patient. And I soon observed the same circumstance. (*London Journal of Medicine.* 1849. i. pp. 54. 976). Some persons indeed, have alleged that the pain of labour can always be prevented, without making the patient unconscious of surrounding objects; whilst others have asserted that no relief can be afforded unless unconsciousness is induced. But both these opinions are directly opposed to experience. There are comparatively few cases in which the suffering can be prevented throughout the labour without interfering with consciousness, although there are very many cases in which it can be in this way pre-vented in the early part of the labour. This difference depends, in some measure, on the constitution of the patient, but chiefly on the severity of the pain to be prevented'[1]. He practised accordingly, for in his diary for 7 April 1853, Snow recorded that chloroform was given to Her Majesty for 53 minutes, in 15 minim doses (= .9ml) dropped on a hand-kerchief. The Queen wrote 'Dr Snow administered that blessed chloroform and the effect was soothing, quieting and delightful beyond measure'.† Chloroform *a la reine* became immediately popular. Snow was never to use the word *analgesia*. Though recorded in the eighteenth century, it seems first to have been used (*analgésie*) in the present sense by Guibert of St Brieuc in 1872[2], who described the state produced by morphine and chloroform.

Apparatus for Analgesia

We have also seen the use of ether/chloroform mixtures by Ellis (p. 214) but the design of specific apparatus for the production of the analgesic state had to wait for a later day. The King Collection possesses two examples, the Minnitt gas/air and the Small ether apparatus, both to be described.

Dr Minnitt gave an account of the history of the development of gas/air analgesia in midwifery in his Presidential Address to the section of Anaesthetics of the Royal Society of Medicine on 1 October 1943[3]. In response to a request from the clinical investigation subcommittee of the Medical Board of the Liverpool Maternity Hospital Minnitt decided that research on nitrous oxide as an analgesic would

---

* Edward Rigby, M.D., Edin. F.R.C.P., (1804–1860), physician to the Lying-In Hospital, Lambeth, and a leading London obstetrician.

† Queen Victoria's diary. April 22, 1853, recording the birth of Prince Leopold. The only record now extant is the copy made by Princess Beatrice after the Queen's death. The originals were then destroyed.

be rewarding. Dr Howard Jones and Dr A.A. Gemmell were involved in the preliminaries, but Dr Minnitt himself, with Charles King, worked out the details: 'on July 19, 1933 I interviewed Mr A. Charles King, then of 34, Devonshire Street, W.1., with regard to a means of employing nitrous oxide inhalations for the relief of labour pains, and we considered the adaptation of a McKesson oxygene thrapy apparatus for the purpose'[3].

McKesson had already attempted the use of seventy per cent nitrous oxide in air; according to Minnitt the unsatisfactory results were due to too high a gas percentage. Within two months Minnitt and Charles King produced the apparatus; the Medical Board of the Liverpool Maternity Hospital, to its great credit, appointed Dr Hilda Garry as research assistant for four months, and the first gas and air analgesia was administered at the hospital on 16 October 1933 (was the day especially chosen, eighty seven years after Morton?). Four days and four cases later, the apparatus was shown in London to the General Meeting of the Association of Anaesthetists of Great Britain and Ireland, and was adopted with great enthusiasm by Dr John Elam of Barnet, who reported upon it in a series of well conceived papers, and produced his own 'carburettor' apparatus: but his report in Liverpool showed his preference for Minnitt's gas/air mixture[4]. Among others who took the idea into their own hospitals were Dr Claude Morris of University College Hospital, Mr Carnac Rivett of Queen Charlotte's Hospital and Dr Katharine Lloyd-Williams of the Royal Free Hospital. The machine and its development are described below.

Analgesia and the Midwives

One other aspect of the analgesia story should be mentioned. At the same meeting of the Association of Anaesthetists, an important resolution was proposed by Dr Howard Jones and seconded by Dr Minnitt. The resolution was amended and resolved thus:

'This general meeting of the Association . . . views with concern any increase in the administration of anaesthetics by unqualified persons, as being a danger to the public, and hopes that if this practice is to be extended to midwives it will only be allowed under strict regulations and after adequate instruction'[5].

Unfortunately the Central Midwives Board later saw fit to insist upon personal medical supervision of midwives using gas/air analgesia, and as Minnitt observed 'the development of the procedure was arrested.' In the meantime the (Royal) College of Obstetricians and Gynaecologists had arranged an investigation of analgesic drugs and methods based on the practice of thirty-six hospitals in the British Isles. A report was published in January 1936, and this paved the way for acceptance by the Central Midwives Board, under strict regulations, of the administration of gas and air by an unsupervised midwife using a recognized apparatus.

As a result of the proportions delivered by Minnitt's machine, it was decided that the specification of an approved apparatus should allow for the delivery of 'not less than fifty five per cent air.' The Minnitt apparatus was thus standardized, and continued to give excellent analgesia, both in domestic and hospital midwifery, up and down the country for many years. It was superseded in the 1950's only when adequate apparatus was designed for the safe use of trichlorethylene[6, 7]. The Tecota, Emotril[8]

FIG. 6.2. MINNITT GAS/AIR
ANALGESIA APPARATUS, 1933.
(Lacking stand, tubing and mask).
The original model, No. 31.
McKesson type reduced pressure
regulator, with intermittent flow
valve. Drum opened to show rubber
reservoir bag. Air is entrained
through a port in the ring above the
pressure gauge. (See Fig. 6.3). This
early model produced 35 per cent
nitrous oxide in air.
CKC 45

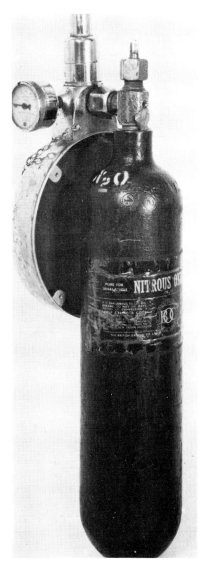

and other apparatus for the production of analgesia
by trichlorethylene are still in the process of making
anaesthetic history, while the turn of the wheel
which has introduced a fifty per cent nitrous
oxide/oxygen analgesic mixture, Entonox, is a story
for the future historian.

CKC 45: MINNITT NITROUS OXIDE/
CKC 45a: AIR ANALGESIA
APPARATUS 1933, 1942

Robert James Minnitt, M.D. (Fig. 6.1) has recently
died after a long working life in Liverpool[9]. The
writer at once acknowledges his friendship and the
gift of a series of reprints relating to the gas/air
apparatus, upon which these notes are largely based.

The original form of the apparatus is that shown
in Figs. 6.2, 6.3. This specimen was manufactured
by Charles King and is numbered 31. It consists of
an adapted McKesson oxygen therapy apparatus,
that is, a reduced pressure regulator attached to a
small rubber bag in a metal drum, an automatic
valve shutting off the flow of gas when the patient
does not inhale. 'The outlet of the machine' wrote
Minnitt, 'is divided into two channels, one for the
passage of gas and one for air, admitted in a constant
amount making a mixture of approximately 35 per
cent nitrous oxide in air'[10].

The face piece is fitted with a spring finger release
which is depressed by the patient during inhalation,
but allows full air if the analgesia becomes deep
enough to weaken the pressure used. The face piece
also has an expiratory valve, and the whole is
attached by a normal fitting to a 100 gallon nitrous
oxide cylinder. Minnitt stated that the average gas
consumption was 35–40 gallons per hour, depending

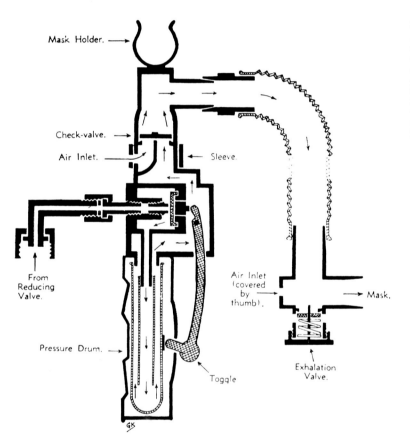

Mask Holder. →

Check-valve. →

Air Inlet. →

Sleeve.

From
Reducing
Valve.

Pressure Drum. →

Toggle

Air Inlet
(covered
by
thumb).

→ Mask.

Exhalation
Valve.

GK

FIG. 6.3. THE MINNITT
APPARATUS,
diagram of original model based on
the McKesson intermittent-flow
valve.
Drawn by Dr Geoffrey Kaye.
From Kaye, G., Orton, S.C.,
Renton, D.G. (1946) *Anaesthetic
Methods*. Melbourne: Ramsay.
p. 377

on the frequency of the 'pains' and depth of breathing. His *Lancet* paper[10] described a series of cases in which electrocardiographic studies and maternal and umbilical vein oxygen content were analysed. The only variation from normal was a reduction in the maternal blood oxygen; umbilical vein blood 'did not show any marked alteration.' The average length of the second stage was within normal limits[11].

Detailed instructions, especially as to the preliminary training of the mother-to-be were given in these and other papers[10, 11, 12].

Reports made by Dr Hilda Garry[13] and Dr John Elam[14], were both greatly encouraging; Dr Minnitt supervised the initial use and the experimental work and became extremely active in pressing for the expansion of the method. The results were described in his paper to the Section of Anaesthetics of the Royal Society of Medicine in August 1934[11], and in 1935 he used gas/air analgesia as an aid in paediatric anaesthesia, a mask with 'traffic lights' being used to engage the attention of the child[15].

Other developments of detail took place. In 1936, the McKesson regulator was replaced by a reservoir bag, 'J' (Fig. 6.4) controlled by a pinchcock, 'I'. Movement of a spring-controlled check valve 'M' in a mixing chamber, brought about by the patient's inspiration, allowed nitrous oxide to flow from the reservoir bag, together with 50 per cent air which was drawn into the mixer through the holes at 'L'; these were of predetermined size and it was stated that constant proportions of nitrous oxide/air were ensured.

Hospital and portable models were produced (Fig. 6.5). By March 1936, four hundred apparatuses were employed in various parts of the world and Dr Minnitt was able to give details of 1,025 deliveries in Liverpool with 'good relief from pain in 952

(92.8%)'[16]. Its use in minor surgery and in dentistry was also mentioned. By 1942, the apparatus fulfilled the delivery need for not less than fifty five per cent air[17], though the final British Oxygen Co. model was set to deliver a constant mixture of 50 per cent air.

One development was described by Minnitt: 'At a meeting of the Section of Obstetrics and Gynaecology (of the Royal Society of Medicine) on 19 Feb. 1937, I was present at the demonstration given by Professor Chassar Moir of a new type of apparatus for the self-administration of nitrous oxide gas during labour (Fig. 6.6). The chief feature in technique was the inhalation of two deep breaths of pure gas before the onset of each pain. Correspondence took place between us in the *British Journal of Anaesthesia* . . . with reference to the relative merits of the two procedures—pure gas *versus* gas and air.

'I conducted some experiments on myself with the help of Dr R.Penn Harbord, Demonstrator in Anaesthesia, University of Liverpool, . . . we found that two or three breaths of pure gas produced the first signs of analgesia in sixteen seconds. This was five to eight seconds quicker than with the standard gas and air machine. In thirty seconds the analgesic effect was most intense: it then declined gradually for fifteen seconds, and became practically absent in sixty seconds. At thirty seconds the gas and air machine produced a state of analgesia as intense as the pure gas, but, of course, this was maintained as long as inhalation continued'[18]. No mention was made of the method of assessing analgesia. Minnitt went on to describe '. . . a special attachment embodying Professor Chassar Moir's suggestion of enabling pure gas to be inhaled from a bag until exhausted (which amounts to two or three deep breaths) . . . and then, as proposed by Dr Elam,

FIG. 6.4. THE MINNITT
APPARATUS
In 1936, the McKesson regulator
was replaced by a reservoir bag,
('J') controlled by pinchcock I. The
spring-loaded check-valve 'M'

allows nitrous oxide to pass to the
patient on inspiration, entraining
50 per cent air through the holes
at 'L'.
Diagram from *British Oxygen
Company* descriptive pamphlet.

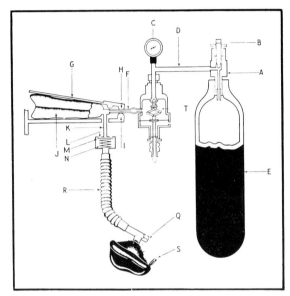

inhalation to be continued with gas and air of the standard percentages.' This special attachment was that produced by the British Oxygen Company and named the *C.M.*★ attachment (Figs. 6.7, 6.8, 6.9). A by-pass 'U' leads gas at one litre per minute from the reservoir bag 'J' to the *C.M.* bag 'W' (Fig. 6.9). The communication between this bag and the face-mask is by way of a diaphragm-operated poppet-valve at 'X'. Negative pressure produced by the patient's inspiration moves the diaphragm which opens the poppet-valve and allows inhalation from bag 'W'. When this bag is exhausted after two or three breaths, the normal Minnitt action of valve 'M' comes into play and the 50 per cent gas/air mixture is inhaled, augmented by the constant flow

★ I am told that the initials *C.M.* are not in any way connected with Professor Chassar Moir. K.B.T.

of 1 litre per minute. In practice this flow reaches the *C.M.* attachment through holes in its inlet tube which match with a notched ring in the Minnitt outlet tube. When the *C.M.* is not attached, this ring is occluded by the corrugated tube mount.

The addition of the *C.M.* attachment invalidated the use of the apparatus by midwives, and the instructions with the machine specifically announce 'The apparatus ceases to conform to the requirements of the Central Midwives Board when this (*C.M.*) attachment is employed. It may, therefore, be used only by a doctor.'

Anoxia?

It is of interest that in the many papers studied, there is no mention of the fact that 55 per cent air contains only 11 per cent oxygen. (But see Kaye, 1946, Fig. 6.3). Warnings against cyanosis are given, especially in 'patients who have an uncompensated heart lesion'[17]; however, in the tables showing oxygen values of maternal and umbilical blood, Minnitt mentions cyanosis occurring in 6 out of 8 mothers, but umbilical values were higher than those of maternal blood and cyanosed mothers did not necessarily produce cyanosed babies[11]. The method therefore was regarded as safe. In a later paper[18], the attachment of a Rowbotham bottle, used with ether, vinyl ether (vinesthene) or trichlorethylene, was described for use by the medical practitioner. In connection with trichlorethylene the statement was made that 'care should be taken that no cyanosis is permitted,' but no indication is given as to how this may be achieved.

In spite of these drawbacks, there is no doubt of the tremendous contribution made by Dr Minnitt to the state of the woman in labour, perhaps the greatest since the days of Simpson. The writer, as a student

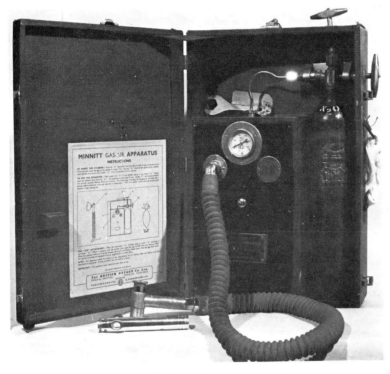

FIG. 6.5. STANDARD MINNITT GAS/AIR APPARATUS, 1939. Originally designed in 1936, this model is identical with that described in Dr Minnitt's presidential paper to the Section of Anaesthetics of the Royal Society of Medicine and designated by him the Queen Charlotte model. The 100 gallon cylinder has a non-removable key; it was filled on 7 December 1951, and still contains gas. The two types of thumb control are shown, one a plain hole, the other spring loaded. The latter had the advantage of shutting off the gas supply, when released. The mask (not shown) had also an expiratory valve. This model has a 'pinchcock' regulator (see Fig. 6.4). CKC 45a

at the time, remembers well the excitement caused by the introduction of the gas/air machine into the maternity department, and the enthusiasm with which it was accepted by the staff, and even more, by the patients.

FIG. 6.6. PROFESSOR CHASSAR MOIR'S APPARATUS
for self-administration of pure nitrous oxide in labour, 1937. This is not in any way related either to the Minnitt apparatus, being based upon the Walton I nitrous oxide machine, or to the *C.M.* attachment, which was designed by the British Oxygen Company for use with the Minnitt apparatus. (Chassar Moir, J. (1937) A New Type of Nitrous Oxide Machine for Self-Induction of Analgesia during Labour. *Proc. Roy. Soc. Med.* **30**, 1281.) The apparatus was manufactured by Charles King.

FIG. 6.7. The *C.M.* nitrous oxide attachment for Minnitt apparatus. Three or four breaths of pure nitrous oxide were available: respiration of nitrous oxide/air then took place.
From a pamphlet issued by the British Oxygen Company. (1952)

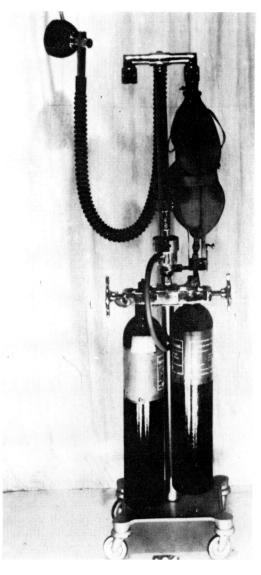

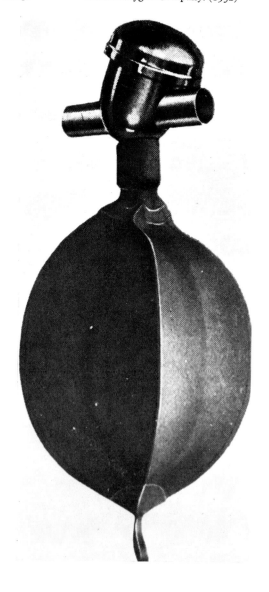

FIG. 6.8. *C.M.* attachment with dome removed to show diaphragm ('V' in Fig. 6.9) and poppet-valve 'X'.
CKC 45b

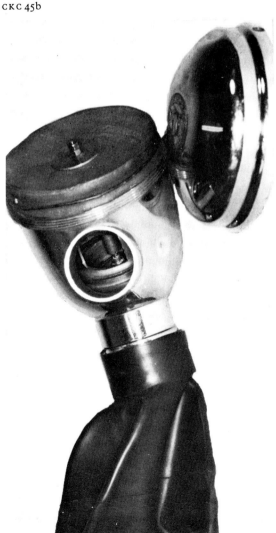

FIG. 6.9. (Cf. Fig. 6.4.). MINNITT APPARATUS WITH *C.M.* ATTACHMENT.
'W' is the reservoir filled at a rate of one litre/minute through tube 'K'. The poppet-valve at 'X' opens when diaphragm 'V' is depressed by inhalation, after reservoir bag is emptied.

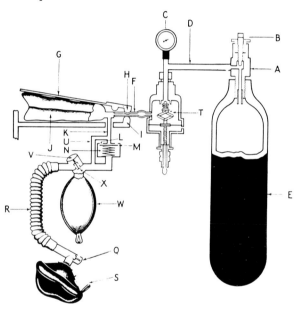

CKC 69: SMALL ETHER ANALGESIA APPARATUS 1937

Dr Thomas H.Small, now retired, still lives in Sydney, where the author has been fortunate in meeting him with his apparatus. The present specimen was presented in 1973 to the Collection, by Dr W.J.Watt, Director of Anaesthetic Services, Auckland Hospital, New Zealand. It carries a New Zealand patent, no. 77610.

The ether container consists of a chromium plated brass drum, 7 in (17.5cm) in diameter and 2 in (5cm) hgih, which holds 10 oz (270cu ml) ether. (Figs. 6.10, 6.11). The mixing valve is on top of the drum, and consists of a ⌣ section rotating tube which uncovers a hole leading to the ether drum; it

FIG. 6.10. Small ether analgesia apparatus, 1937, in carrying box. Photograph by Dr Thomas Small of the example used at the Royal Hospital for Women, Sydney, and shown to the author in 1972. In this specimen, the ether/air mixing valve is mounted to the side of the ether drum. (Cf. Fig. 6.11.) Sometimes trichlorethylene was substituted for ether.

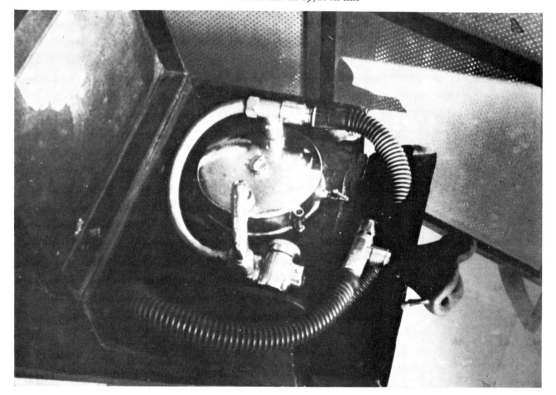

also communicates with the conical efferent tube on the opposite side, as the control is opened. This cone has a one-way flap valve leading to the red rubber spirally wound elephant tube, and there is another one-way inspiratory flap in the opening of the mixing valve. The mask is by Heidbrink, and the angle-piece has an expiratory valve with a fixed spring control.

The apparatus does not seem to have been described by Dr Small, but in a paper reporting a meeting of Australian obstetricians[19] in 1937, he discussed its use, and other participants commented favourably upon it. Small reported that various authorities including Dr Katharine Lloyd Williams, advocated ether in obstetrics; however she said that analgesia was slow in onset and generally coincided with the first stage of anaesthesia. Dr Small found that ether analgesia was a definite stage preceding loss of consciousness. He recorded two hundred cases from the Royal Hospital for Women, Sydney. Analgesia was obtained if one-sixteenth to one-eighth of the inspired air passed over the ether,

FIG. 6.11. Small ether analgesia apparatus.
The mixing valve is mounted on top of the ether drum. The opening has a brass inspiratory flap valve. A flap valve also is placed in the cone shaped efferent tube, and a separate expiratory valve on the angle-piece to the celluloid Heidbrink face piece. The ether filler is to the right and the ether/air control at the further end of the mixing valve.
CKC 69

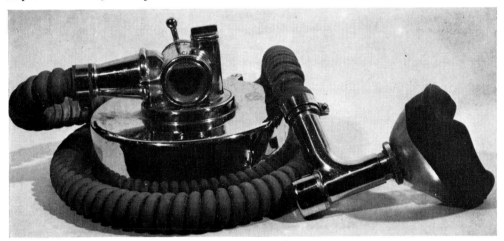

and the apparatus used one and a half ounces (40 cu ml) of ether per hour, the strength of the vapour at one eighth being three per cent. The parturient could administer it herself, and in discussion, Dr S.V.Marshall considered it safer in this context than the Minnitt apparatus, which produced annoxaemia. Dr Hunter of Sydney said that this machine was very safe, while administration of nitrous oxide and oxygen required a trained anaesthetist.

This piece of apparatus is of particular interest in that ether has never been generally considered suitable for analgesic purposes, few references to this property occurring in the literature of ether. This apparatus seems to have been confined in its use to the Antipodes, but Dr Small has said that it was in use until recently in Sydney, trichlorethylene being occasionally substituted for diethyl ether.

REFERENCES

1 SNOW J. (1858) *On Chloroform and other Anaesthetics.* London: Churchill. p. 318.

2 DUNCUM B. (1947) *Development of Inhalation Anaesthesia.* London: Oxford Univ. Press. p. 380 Appendix B.

3 MINNITT R.J. (1944) The History and Progress of Gas and Air Analgesia for Midwifery. *Proc. Roy. Soc. Med.* **37.** 45.

4 ELAM J. (1934) *Report on the Investigation of Gas and Air Analgesia in Midwifery, Carried out at the Wellhouse Hospital, Barnet.* In Minnitt, R.J., *Self Administered Analgesia for the Midwifery of General Practice.* read at the Liverpool Medical Institution, 22 February 1934.

5 FEATHERSTONE H.W. (1951) *The Association of Anaesthetists of Great Britain and Ireland. Notes on its inception and earlier activities.* Typescript from the Minute Books (1932–40) of the Association.

6 FREEDMAN A. (1943) Trichlorethylene-air Analgesia in Childbirth. An investigation with a suitable inhaler. *Lancet* **ii.** 696.

7 SEWARD E.H. (1949) Self administered analgesia in labour with special reference to trichlorethylene. *Lancet.* **ii.** 781.

8 EPSTEIN H.G., & MACINTOSH R.R. (1949) Analgesia Inhaler for Trichlorethylene. *Brit. med. J.* **ii.** 1092.

9 Obituary notice: (1974) Robert James Minnitt. *Brit. med. J.* **i.** 464.

10 MINNITT R.J. (1934) A New Technique for the Self-Administration of Gas-Air Analgesia in Labour. *Lancet.* **i.** 1278.

11 MINNITT, R.J. (1934) Self-Administered Analgesia for the Midwifery of General Practice. *Proc. Roy. Soc. Med.* **27.** (*Sect. Anaesth.*) p. 1313.

12 MINNITT R.J. (1934) *The Minnitt Gas-Air Analgesia Apparatus for the Midwifery of General Practice.* Research notes presented at the meeting of the Royal Society of Medicine (Anaesthetic Section), 4 May 1934.

13 GARRY HILDA (1934) Report to Liverpool Medical Institution on the *Investigation of Gas and Air Analgesia in Midwifery.* 22 Feb. 1934.

14 ELAM J. (1934) *Report on Investigation of Gas and Air Analgesia in Midwifery . . .* at the Wellhouse Hospital, Barnet. Read to Liverpool Medical Institution. 22 Feb. 1934.

15 MINNITT R.J. (1935) Gas-Air Analgesia as an aid to Anaesthesia in Children. *Liverpool Med. Chir. J.* **43.** 120.

16 MINNITT R.J. (1936) Gas and Air Analgesia: Obstetrical-Surgical-Dentistry. *Liverpool Med. Chir. J.* **44.** 102.

17 MINNITT R.J. (1942) Analgesia and Anaesthesia in Midwifery. *Med. Press.* p. 208.

18 MINNITT R.J. (1944) The History and Progress of Gas and Air Analgesia for Midwifery. (Presidential Address). *Proc. Roy. Soc. Med.* **37.** 45.

19 SMALL T.H. (1937) Ether Analgesia and Analgesia in Midwifery. *Medical J. Australia.* **10.** (3). 708–709.

Section VII
Face Masks and Drop-Methods

ILLUSTRATIONS

Frontispiece. Book plate of Charles King. (Courtesy of the Librarian, Royal Society of Medicine, London).

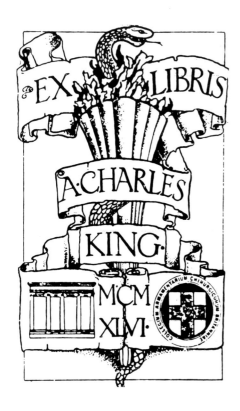

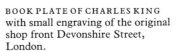

BOOK PLATE OF CHARLES KING
with small engraving of the original
shop front Devonshire Street,
London.
From the copy of Edward Murphy
On Chloroform, 1855, (see p. 67),
now in the library of the Royal
Society of Medicine.

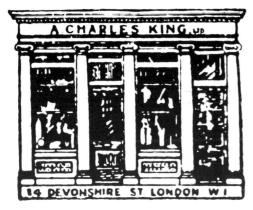

INTRODUCTION: *MORTON SUBSTITUTES A SPONGE*

The use of ether in an 'open' manner dates from the early days. In 1847, the ether-soaked bell-shaped sponge had become popular and was described by no less an authority than Morton himself. In June 1847 in the *Lancet* letter already quoted (p. 7), Morton wrote 'I was never satisfied with any apparatus at all for the purpose of inhalation, there being so much repugnance to it. I was led, therefore, to make further experiments on this subject, which have resulted in an entire abandonment of my old inhaler, and the substitution of the sponge'[1]. This is an interesting remark, which does not appear previously to have been noticed. The Editor of the *Lancet* in a note to the letter pointed out that Dr Thomas Smith of Cheltenham had for some time recommended this method. Smith had used it in 1847 in probably the first description of an *examination under anaesthesia*, in a child of two suffering from ophthalmia[2].

The introduction of chloroform, in Britain at least, led to a relative abandonment of ether, though in America it was not long before John Collins Warren was writing from the Massachusetts General Hospital, recommending 'the return to ether', which he used 'freely in a sponge or cloth'[3]. Simpson used 'the corner of a towel' for administering chloroform (Fig. 7.1) while Lister followed the teaching of his father-in-law, James Syme, 1799–1870, that 'every case was one for chloroform.' In 1861, Lister wrote— 'a common towel being arranged so as to form a

FIG. 7.1. SIMPSON'S METHOD of administering chloroform on the corner of a towel.

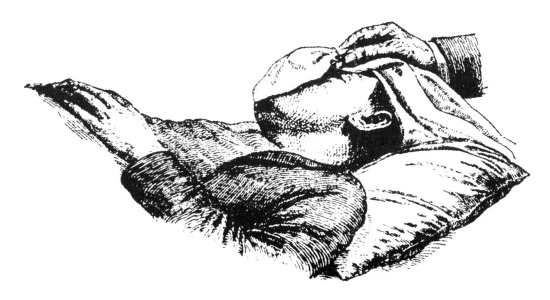

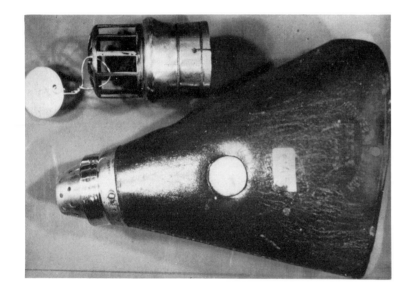

FIG. 7.2. HYDERABAD 'CONE',
1890.
The hole in the leather cone
admitted air and chloroform. The
expiratory 'cage' (separated)
contained a feather respiratory
indicator.
From Geoffrey Kaye Museum,
Melbourne. No. J(2) 4.

square cloth of six folds, enough chloroform is poured on it to moisten a surface in the middle about as large as the palm of the hand, the precise quantity being a matter of no consequence whatever . . . the cloth is held as near the face as can comfortably be borne, more chloroform being added as may be necessary'[4]. Later, Lister was to use Simpson's single layer; his students (who gave the chloroform) were taught a series of rules which included the aphorism 'Towel versus engines. Brains versus valves'[5].

Simpson's towel was soon pinned up into a cone with a small sponge in its apex, and both *Rendle's mask, c.* 1870, (p. 43) and Edward Lawrie's *Hydera-bad cone* of 1890 (Fig. 7.2) followed this idea. All these limited oxygen and allowed accumulation of carbon dioxide in a manner which must be considered dangerous, particularly when using chloroform.

THE MASKS IN THE KING COLLECTION

Thus it was some twenty years before the wire mask appeared, the first being that of Thomas Skinner, d. 1906, obstetric physician to the Liverpool Dispensary. Like Snow, Skinner was interested in cholera, but, unlike Snow, he was also a homeo-pathist[6]. He described his mask in 1862[7]; it was much used in Europe, and was recommended by Probyn-Williams as late as 1909[8].

Skinner's paper gave details of the *pros and cons* of the use of chloroform in labour, and he recognized the 'special tolerance for chloroform in midwifery, which does not pertain to the practice of surgery'. The mask (CKC 50, Fig. 7.3) consists of a circular wire frame 14cm in diameter; a second wire holds the single layer of lint or flannel some 5 or 6cm from

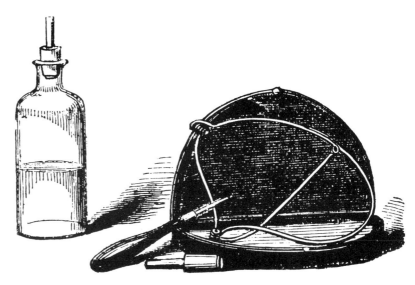

FIG. 7.3. SKINNER'S
CHLOROFORM MASK, 1862.
From *British Medical Journal*.
(1862) **ii**, 110.
The whole wire frame, and the
handle, fold flat for carrying.
Cf. CKC 50

the face, and a handle is provided. The whole folds flat, in order that it may be carried in the top hat. The mask still appeared in the catalogues in 1925 (cost 4/6) and 1938 (7/6). Skinner also described a simple drop-bottle for use with his mask.

In 1868, John Murray, 1844–1873, produced a wedge-shaped wire mask, which carried several layers of flannel, stated to absorb from one-half to one drachm (2.5ml) of chloroform. Murray's paper described 'an aperture in the cover for the admission of air, which however, may, if necessary, be also allowed to enter at the sides'[9]. The mask folded, and fitted with a graduated bottle, into a case. (CKC 51, Fig. 7.4).

John Murray (Fig. 7.5) was chloroformist and later, assistant physician, to the Middlesex Hospital. He was evidently a brilliant young man, who died young, his bust being subsequently placed in the museum at his hospital[10].

The change to ether had been advocated in 1877 by the distinguished Swiss surgeon, Gustave Julliard, 1836–1911[11], who had been virtually the founder of the medical faculty in Geneva. In 1871, Julliard had a patient who suffered a fatal cardiac arrest when using chloroform for the reduction of a dislocated shoulder. A subsequent near-fatality made him lose confidence in the drug, and he described in a later paper[12] the change to ether in which he carried with him many Continental colleages. The present mask (Figs. 7.4, 7.6, 7.7) was also described, with a drawing, and at a French Congress in 1902, he claimed no deaths in 9289 ether administrations. The mask became very popular, and Julliard gave the following conditions for its design: 1. the exterior should be covered with an impermeable material to prevent loss of ether vapour. 2. the mask should be large enough not to suffocate the patient; at least 15cm by 12cm by

FIG. 7.4. Wire-frame masks from the Charles King Collection.
Murray, No. 51, 1868.
Julliard, No. 9, 1877.
Schimmelbusch, No. 68, 1890.

Kocher, No. 49, c. 1890.
Tyrrell, No. 52, c. 1890.
Yankauer, No. 54, 1910.
Low, No. 53, c. 1910.

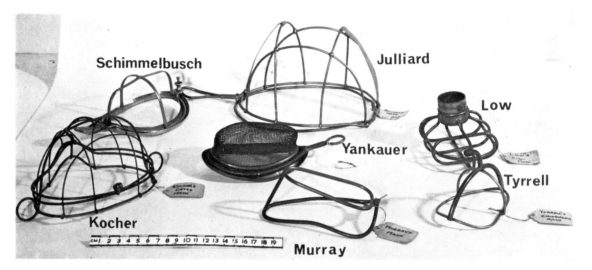

15cm in height. These measurements are borne out by the Charles King Collection specimen. Julliard stated that he had himself been anaesthetized on two occasions with his own mask, and he made an italic demand that the ether should always be given by *'une personne capable qui ne fera que cela et qui ne s'occupera que de cela.'* Julliard's mask, if used as he intended, must have offered a bonus to hypoxia, while allowing accumulation of carbon dioxide.

Seven wire masks of various periods from the Collection are shown in Fig. 7.4. Of these the generic and eponymic pattern is that of Kurt Schimmelbusch, 1860–1895, of Berlin. Duncum[13] quotes a German reference of 1890 for the appearance of this mask, the only one whose name is known to all anaesthetists. By this time, both chloroform and ether were dripped on to lint or flannel, the same wire frame being used for both drugs, and for their mixtures, such as the A.C.E. of Harley, 1860, (p. 211) or McCardie's unusual

$C_1 E_{16}$[14]. The Schimmelbusch mask (CKC 68) was the first to be specially designed for any of these, the trough-like rim being arranged to catch surplus fluid. When used for chloroform, one layer of lint was general, while for ether up to six or eight layers of gauze were customary. It was also usual to cover the mask, when using ether, with a split piece of gauze to prevent evaporation, a technique still in vogue. Sometimes a waxed outer cover served this purpose, though this was more commonly a continental practice, following Julliard. Of the other masks shown in Fig. 7.4, that of Theodore Kocher, 1841–1917, Professor of Surgery at Berne, was in use about 1890. It consists of a hemispherical wire basket of about 15cm diameter, used with a gauze cover. In his *Textbook*[15], Kocher wrote a chapter on anaesthesia in which he asked 'why not put chloroform aside?' He described a large ether and smaller chloroform masks, preferring the drop method to the use of Junker's inhaler, and he

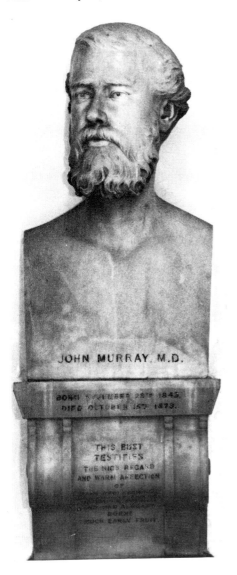

FIG. 7.5. JOHN MURRAY, 1844–1873.
Commemorative bust at the Middlesex Hospital, London.

JOHN MURRAY, M.D.

BORN SEPTEMBER 29TH 1845.
DIED OCTOBER 1ST 1873.

THIS BUST
TESTIFIES
THE HIGH REGARD
AND WARM AFFECTION
OF

recommended for the patient a cup of tea with cognac half an hour before the anaesthetic, to strengthen the heart's action, and raise the blood pressure.

Yankauer's mask (CKC 54, Fig. 7.4) is assigned to 1910, and was designed by Sidney Yankauer, (d. 1932) of the Mount Sinai Hospital, New York, a pioneer bronchoscopist. His mask consists of an oval wire mesh, 13cm by 9cm, with a handle, and was described by Gwathmey in 1914 as one of the best masks for the drop method of ether or chloroform[16]. Gwathmey himself modified the Yankauer mask by fashioning the rim out of a hollow tube through which oxygen could be passed. This is still in use in America. In *Down Brothers'* catalogue of 1938 Yankauer's mask was priced at seven shillings and sixpence.

The ether masks of Walter Tyrrell, 1852–1931, the first anaesthetist appointed to St Thomas's Hospital[17] (*c.* 1880) and of Harold Low, *c.* 1865–1932, his pupil, of the same hospital, are also shown in Fig. 7.4. That of Tyrrell, (CKC 52) about 1890, is a simple wire frame with a hollow raised central bar for the passage of oxygen. The *Surgical Manufacturers Catalogue* for 1925 offers Tyrrell's mask for eight shillings and sixpence. Tyrrell was better known for his ingenious modification of the Junker apparatus in which ether was used with chloroform, described in a paper read to the Society of Anaesthetists in 1897[18], the Society which later (1905) became the Section of Anaesthetics of the Royal Society of Medicine.

Harold Low was appointed to the staff of St Thomas's Hospital in 1895[19]. His mask does not seem to have been described.* It consists of a small

* Harold Low's mask was wrongly ascribed in my Invenory to Dr Alexander Low, also of St Thomas' Hospital. K.B.T.

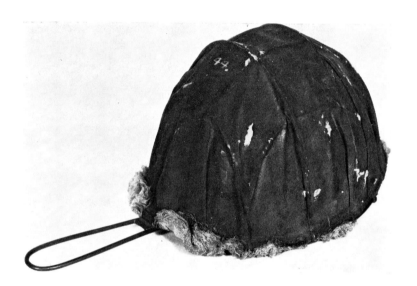

FIG. 7.6. JULLIARD ETHER MASK, 1877.
The impermeable outer cover is shown. (Cf. Fig. 7.4.).
This is a complete specimen from the Collection of the Royal College of Surgeons of England.

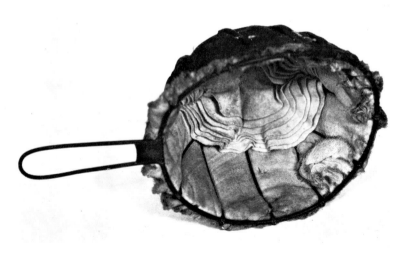

FIG. 7.7. INTERIOR OF THE JULLIARD MASK,
to show 'rosette' of flannel, on to which 20–25ml ether was poured for induction, similar doses being subsequently applied.

FIG. 7.8. LOW ETHER MASK,
c. 1910.
An unusual design in having a collar for a face mask. The cage was covered with 6–8 layers of gauze.
CKC 53

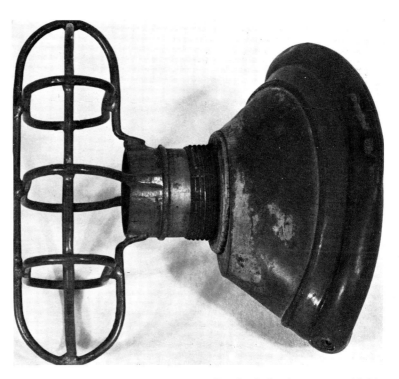

ovoid wire frame, and is unusual in having a collar for a face mask. It would seem that the anaesthetist would receive as much ether as the patient. (CKC 53, Fig. 7.8). A contemporary colleague, Dr John Ryan, writes 'As far as I know the mask was the only piece of apparatus he (Low) invented. He used it for induction as well as maintenance. It (ether) was dripped from a bottle on to the 6–8 layers of gauze. . . . The induction was a very slow process as the average patient found it difficult to tolerate a concentration sufficiently high for much progress to be made. There was a lot of coughing, laryngeal spasm and a prolonged and often boisterous excite-

ment stage. . . . Low's inductions were highly thought of by the surgical dressers, providing, as they did, some light relief. . . . The mask was quite a good way of maintaining anaesthesia . . . with the inflatable cuff on the face-mask a good fit could be obtained and so one had a semiclosed system and a high concentration of ether could be built up'[20]. Low conducted active general practice in Chelsea, devoting his mornings to this and to private anaesthesia, and the afternoon sessions to his hospital work. He was appointed anaesthetist to the Royal family after anaesthetizing the Duchess of Connaught upon two occasions.

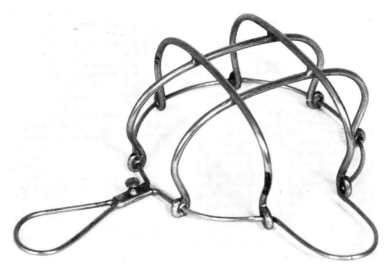

FIG. 7.9. MCCARDIE ETHER MASK,
1900.
CKC A5

The mask described by William John McCardie, 1865–1939, of Birmingham, consists of a stout wire frame, about 10 × 10 × 5cm with a handle; multiple layers of gauze were used (Fig. 7.9). McCardie was the first provincial full-time anaesthetist, who introduced ethyl chloride into this country in 1901, and who wrote many papers on anaesthetic matters. He was also to produce a double-ended ether inhaler, for adults and children.

INHALERS

The examples shown in Fig. 7.10 may be described as 'open inhalers', rather than masks, since they contain a sponge or gauze within an enclosed area, and so tend to allow a greater amount of rebreathing than is possible with most 'open masks'.

Those of Silk, 1893, (CKC 64) Denis Browne, (CKC 62) and Flagg, 1939 (CKCA2) have already been described (pp. 43, 47, 49). The inhaler attributed by Charles King to Alexander Ogston, 1844–1929, Professor of Surgery in Aberdeen, is numbered Aust.19. It consists of an oval wire frame about 15 × 6 × 8cm in depth, with intermediate wires, about 1cm apart, which were interleaved with gauze. This was an obvious attempt to copy and modify the inhaler of O.H.Allis of Philadelphia, first demonstrated in 1874; Allis's was the first American 'open' inhaler (Fig. 7.11); as the wire cage was surrounded by a leather jacket, a considerable amount of rebreathing took place. Nonetheless this was an early attempt to break away from the system of air-restriction advocated by those who used a rebreathing bag (as in the Clover inhaler), and Allis's inhaler was influential in America in the move away from such methods. On the Continent at the same time, came modifications of Skinner's mask made by Friedrich von Esmarch, which in the 1880's was most commonly used for the administration of

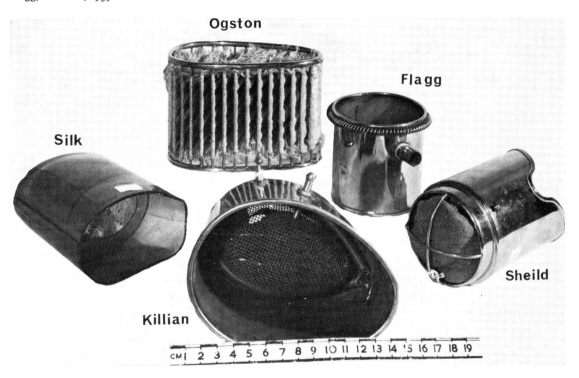

chloroform.

Fig. 7.10 also shows the open inhaler of Marmaduke Sheild, 1850–1922, of St George's Hospital, and that of Gustav Killian, 1860–1921, the introducer of direct laryngoscopy. References to his mask have not been found.

Sheild's (CKC A4) consists of a circular metal face mask 13cm deep, shaped to nose and mouth. Two sponges at the distal end are retained by a hinged wire flap. This inhaler would seem to suffer from most of the drawbacks complained of in contemporary literature, particularly those arising from cooling of the ether, and of saturating the exhaled air to the discomforture of surgeon, anaesthetist and nurse. Sheild was particularly interested in the teaching of anaesthetists and wrote a paper advocating its incorporation in the medical curriculum[21].

Killian's inhaler, No. Aust. 6., dated to 1900, consists of an ovoid metal frame some 15cm high, with a wire mesh and a spring lint retainer about 6cm from the patient's face. There is an oxygen inlet below the lint and three hooks are provided for a rubber harness, probably the earliest of this type to appear.

It is noteworthy that many of these masks and inhalers appeared in the years around 1900. This

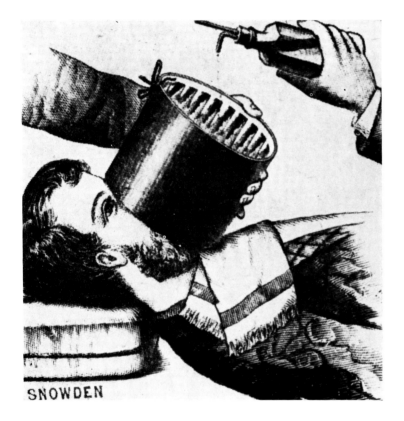

FIG. 7.11. ALLIS ETHER INHALER, 1874.

SNOWDEN

was a time when the chloroform controversy was at its height[22], and when some anaesthetists, particularly in America, were beginning to suspect that the oxygen restriction offered by the 'open' inhaler was not necessarily in the patient's best interests. As late as 1928, Denis Browne wrote of Silk's inhaler 'the sponge, however, when soaked with ether, is almost impermeable to air. . .'[23]. It is also notable that, in 1907, so important an anaesthetist as H.E.G.Boyle was describing the administration of chloroform by drop, using only a double thickness of lint held over the face[24].

For these reasons we see attempts to add oxygen inlet tubes to some of these pieces. Of them all only the Schimmelbusch has survived to the present day, though it is difficult to find any explanation as to why this particular mask should have done so. Its early popularity seems to have been due to the fact that it was the first to supply a gutter to prevent overspill from reaching the patient's face, an item also incorporated in the popular American mask of Yankaeur.

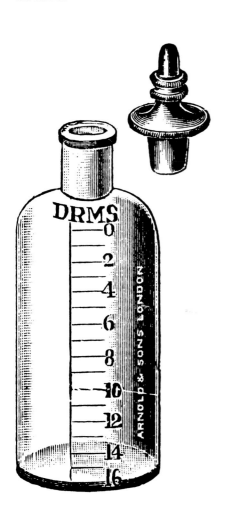

DROP-BOTTLES

With the rag came the bottle; almost every anaesthetist had his own pattern, but only two are
represented in the King Collection, one being for
chloroform and one for ether.

Joseph Mills, d. 1893, was the first full-time
anaesthetist to St Bartholomew's Hospital from
1875–1893. His bottle for chloroform was described
about 1880, and also by Boyle in 1907 (CKC 10,
Fig. 7.12). This was literally a 'drop' bottle, one
shake producing one drop and twenty drops being
equivalent to about 1 drachm. (= 3.4ml).

Jackson, of the Evelina Children's Hospital, described his ether bottle in 1914[25] (CKC 59) as consisting of a large pear shaped bottle of 200ml
capacity, (Fig. 7.13), with a fine pouring tube and a
tap. The air inlet in the tap is so arranged that ether
runs slowly only when the bottle is tilted, even though
the tap is open. This bottle appears to have had a
vogue, as it is described both by Dudley Buxton in
1914[26] and by Blomfield in 1917[27]. Jackson's
original paper shows the flask held in a 'restful position' in one hand, the index and middle fingers
operating a 'rudder' attached to the tap, from which
ether can be dripped 'at any pace from ten drops to
the minute upwards'. This is not present on the
present example, which has a small air inlet above
the tap, allowing control by a finger.

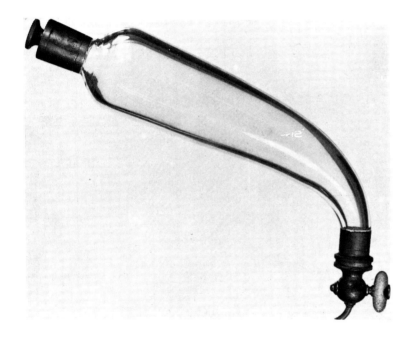

FIG. 7.13. JACKSON ETHER DROP-
BOTTLE, 1914.
The flange on the tap has an air
hole, which may be controlled by
the finger.
CKC 59

REFERENCES

1 MORTON W.T.G. (1847) Letter from Dr Morton of Boston. *Lancet.* **ii.** 80.

2 SMITH T. (1847) Remarks on the Inhalation of Ether. *London Medical Gaz.* **5** (*n.s.*). 676.

3 WARREN J.C. (1849) Effects of choloform and strong chloric ether. *London Medical Gaz.* **8.** (*n.s.*). 757.

4 LISTER J. (1909) *The Collected Papers of Joseph Baron Lister.* Oxford: Clarendon Press. Vol. **I.** p. 143.

5 TURNBULL L. (1892) Chloroform Administration in Edinburgh. *Brit. Med. J.* **ii.** 936.

6 Obituary notice: (1906) Dr Thomas Skinner. *Homeopathic World.* (London). **41.** 418.

7 SKINNER T. (1862) Anaesthesia in Midwifery: with new apparatus for its safer induction by choloform. *Brit Med. J.* **ii.** 108.

8 PROBYN-WILLIAMS R.J. (1909) *Practical Guide to the Administration of Anaesthetics.* London: Longmans, Green, 2nd ed. p. 150.

9 [MURRAY J.] (1868) Chloroform Inhaler of Dr John Murray. *Medical Times and Gazette.* **i.** 540.

10 Editorial note (1874) Memorial bust of the late Dr John Murray. *Brit. Med. J.* **ii.** 118.

11 Obituary notice: (1911) *Revue médicale de la Suisse romande.* **31.** 659.

12 JULLIARD G. (1891) L'éther est-il préférable au chloroforme?

Revue médicale de la Suisse romande. **11.** 81–128.

13 DUNCUM B. (1947) *The Development of Inhalation Anaesthesia.* London: Oxford Univ. Press. p. 252.

14 McCARDIE W.J. (1917) A Method of Anaesthetizing Soldiers. *Brit. Med. J.* **i.** 508.

15 KOCHER T. (1895) *Textbook of Operative Surgery.* trans. Stiles. London: Black.

16 GWATHMEY J.T. (1914) *Anesthesia.* New York: Appleton. p. 203.

17 Obituary notice: (1931) Walter Tyrrell. *Brit. Med. J.* **i.** 826.

18 TYRRELL W. (1898) On the addition of ether vapour from a Second Bottle during Chloroform Administration by Junker Apparatus. *Trans. Soc. Anaesth.* **i.** 1.

19 Obituary notice: (1932) (Harold Low). *Brit. J. Anaesth.* **10.** 44.

20 Dr John Ryan to Dr Charles Foster, St. Thomas's Hospital London. (Courtesy of Dr Ryan and Dr Foster.)

21 SHEILD M. (1896) The Neglect of Teaching in Anaesthetics. *Practitioner.* **57.** 387.

22 THOMAS K.B. (1974) Chloroform: Commissions and Omissions. *Proc. Roy. Soc. Med.* **67.** 723–730.

23 BROWNE D. (1928) Anaesthesia for Tonsillectomy. . . . *Brit. Med. J.* **ii.** 632.

24 BOYLE H.E.G. (1907) *Practical Anaesthetics.* London. Hodder

and Stoughton. p. 90.

25 JACKSON D. (1913) A New Ether Drop Bottle. *Lancet.* **ii.** 1779.

26 BUXTON D.W. (1914) *Anaesthetics.* London. Lewis. 5th ed. p. 161.

27 BLOMFIELD J. (1917) *Anaesthetics.* London. Baillière, Tindall and Cox. 4th ed. p. 47.

Index